OTHER *FAST FACTS* BOOKS

Fast Facts on ADOLESCENT HEALTH FOR NURSING AND HEALTH PROFESSIONALS: A Care Guide (*Herrman*)

Fast Facts for the ADULT-GERONTOLOGY ACUTE CARE NURSE PRACTITIONER (*Carpenter*)

Fast Facts for the ANTEPARTUM AND POSTPARTUM NURSE: A Nursing Orientation and Care Guide (*Davidson*)

Fast Facts Workbook for CARDIAC DYSRHYTHMIAS AND 12-LEAD EKGs (*Desmarais*)

Fast Facts for the CARDIAC SURGERY NURSE: Caring for Cardiac Surgery Patients, Third Edition (*Hodge*)

Fast Facts for CAREER SUCCESS IN NURSING: Making the Most of Mentoring (*Vance*)

Fast Facts for the CATH LAB NURSE, Second Edition (*McCulloch*)

Fast Facts for the CLASSROOM NURSING INSTRUCTOR: Classroom Teaching (*Yoder-Wise, Kowalski*)

Fast Facts for the CLINICAL NURSE LEADER (*Wilcox, Deerhake*)

Fast Facts for the CLINICAL NURSE MANAGER: Managing a Changing Workplace, Second Edition (*Fry*)

Fast Facts for the CLINICAL NURSING INSTRUCTOR: Clinical Teaching, Third Edition (*Kan, Stabler-Haas*)

Fast Facts on COMBATING NURSE BULLYING, INCIVILITY, AND WORKPLACE VIOLENCE: What Nurses Need to Know (*Ciocco*)

Fast Facts About COMPETENCY-BASED EDUCATION IN NURSING: How to Teach Competency Mastery (*Wittmann-Price, Gittings*)

Fast Facts for the CRITICAL CARE NURSE, Second Edition (*Hewett*)

Fast Facts About CURRICULUM DEVELOPMENT IN NURSING: How to Develop and Evaluate Educational Programs, Second Edition (*McCoy, Anema*)

Fast Facts for DEMENTIA CARE: What Nurses Need to Know, Second Edition (*Miller*)

Fast Facts for DEVELOPING A NURSING ACADEMIC PORTFOLIO: What You Really Need to Know (*Wittmann-Price*)

Fast Facts About DIVERSITY, EQUITY, AND INCLUSION IN NURSING: Building Competencies for an Antiracism Practice (*Davis*)

Fast Facts for DNP ROLE DEVELOPMENT: A Career Navigation Guide (*Menonna-Quinn, Tortorella Genova*)

Fast Facts About EKGs FOR NURSES: The Rules of Identifying EKGs (*Landrum*)

Fast Facts for the ER NURSE: Guide to a Successful Emergency Department Orientation, Fourth Edition (*Buettner*)

Fast Facts for EVIDENCE-BASED PRACTICE IN NURSING, Third Edition (*Godshall*)

Fast Facts for the FAITH COMMUNITY NURSE: Implementing FCN/Parish Nursing (*Hickman*)

Fast Facts About FORENSIC NURSING: What You Need to Know (*Scannell*)

Fast Facts on GENETICS AND GENOMICS FOR NURSES: Practical Applications (*Subasic*)

Fast Facts for the GERONTOLOGY NURSE: A Nursing Care Guide (*Eliopoulos*)

Fast Facts About GI AND LIVER DISEASES FOR NURSES: What APRNs Need to Know (*Chaney*)

Fast Facts About the GYNECOLOGICAL EXAM: A Professional Guide for NPs, PAs, and Midwives, Second Edition (*Secor, Fantasia*)

Fast Facts in HEALTH INFORMATICS FOR NURSES (*Hardy*)

Fast Facts for HEALTH PROMOTION IN NURSING: Promoting Wellness (*Miller*)

Fast Facts for Nurses About HOME INFUSION THERAPY: The Expert's Best Practice Guide (*Gorski*)

Fast Facts for the HOSPICE NURSE: A Concise Guide to End-of-Life Care, Second Edition (*Wright*)

Fast Facts for the L&D NURSE: Labor & Delivery Orientation, Third Edition (*Groll*)

Fast Facts About LGBTQ+ CARE FOR NURSES (*Traister*)

Fast Facts for the LONG-TERM CARE NURSE: What Nursing Home and Assisted Living Nurses Need to Know (*Eliopoulos*)

Fast Facts to LOVING YOUR RESEARCH PROJECT: A Stress-Free Guide for Novice Researchers in Nursing and Healthcare (*Marshall*)

Fast Facts for MAKING THE MOST OF YOUR CAREER IN NURSING (*Redulla*)

Fast Facts for MANAGING PATIENTS WITH A PSYCHIATRIC DISORDER: What RNs, NPs, and New Psych Nurses Need to Know (*Marshall*)

Fast Facts About MEDICAL CANNABIS AND OPIOIDS: Minimizing Opioid Use Through Cannabis (*Smith, Smith*)

Fast Facts for the MEDICAL OFFICE NURSE: What You Really Need to Know (*Richmeier*)

Fast Facts for the MEDICAL–SURGICAL NURSE: Clinical Orientation (*Ciocco*)

Fast Facts for the OPERATING ROOM NURSE, Third Edition (*Criscitelli*)

Fast Facts for PATIENT SAFETY IN NURSING: How to Decrease Medical Errors and Improve Patient Outcomes (*Hunt*)

Fast Facts for PSYCHOPHARMACOLOGY FOR NURSE PRACTITIONERS (*Goldin*)

Fast Facts for the SCHOOL NURSE, Fourth Edition (*Loschiavo*)

Fast Facts About STROKE CARE FOR THE ADVANCED PRACTICE NURSE (*Morrison*)

FAST FACTS

About

STROKE CARE FOR THE ADVANCED PRACTICE NURSE

Kathy J. Morrison, MSN, RN, SCRN, FAHA, is a certified stroke nurse, a Fellow of the American Heart Association, and a recipient of the prestigious Pennsylvania State Nightingale Award for Clinical Nursing Excellence. As the stroke program manager for the Penn State Hershey Medical Center, she oversaw all aspects of stroke care, from prehospital through stroke clinic follow-up, until her retirement in 2021. She played a pivotal role in Penn State Hershey Medical Center's attainment of The Joint Commission Comprehensive Stroke Center (CSC) certification, and has mentored many stroke program coordinators through the process of attaining Primary and CSC certification. Ms. Morrison also served on The Joint Commission Expert Panel for Stroke Center certification standards.

Ms. Morrison's published works have appeared in nursing journals and neuroscience course curricula. Her books *Fast Facts for Stroke Care Nursing* First and Second Editions, *Stroke Certification Study Guide for Nurses, and Stroke Nursing Certification Review* have been well received in the nursing community, both as handy guides for stroke care nurses and as preparation tools for the SCRN® certification exam. Even in retirement, she remains active in leading SCRN review courses, participating in community stroke awareness campaigns, and facilitating a regional stroke survivor support group. She established the Stroke Coordinators of Pennsylvania (SCoPA) in 2010—a group of stroke coordinators whose collaborative work has resulted in significant improvements in stroke care and outcomes in community hospitals across central Pennsylvania. She is a Fellow of the American Heart Association, a member of the American Association of Neuroscience Nurses, a board member of the Susquehanna Valley Chapter of the American Association of Neuroscience Nurses, and a board member of the Stroke Survivors Foundation.

Diane McLaughlin, DNP, AGACNP-BC, CCRN, FCCM, FNCS, is an acute care nurse practitioner at Baptist Medical Center/Lyerly Neurosurgery and Mayo Clinic Florida. She specializes in the field of neurocritical care and is a world expert and international speaker on topics such as stroke, advanced practice provider (APP) training, and point-of-care ultrasound. She is active in healthcare, a recent chair of the APP Resource Committee for the Society of Critical Care Medicine (SCCM), and chair-elect for the Advanced Practice Nursing Professional Development Committee of the Nursing Section, as well as serving on strategic planning, congress program planning, and ultrasound committees. She was recently accepted into the American College of Critical Care Medicine as a Fellow of Critical Care Medicine, which is a designation honoring practitioners who have made outstanding contributions in critical care. Dr. McLaughlin is a member of the Neurocritical Care Society Guidelines and APP Leadership committees, and serves as a social media ambassador for the journal *Neurocritical Care*. She was also inducted as a Fellow of Neurocritical Care in 2022. She is passionate about APP training and is a part-time lecturer at Case Western Reserve University. She spends much of her free time helping to advance the role of the critical care APP at the bedside. She is knowledgeable in research and academia, and has authored many publications, presentations, and book chapters, including the book *Fast Facts About Neurocritical Care for Nurse Practitioners and Physician Assistants*. She is dedicated to the advancement of science and healing the sick.

FAST FACTS

About

STROKE CARE FOR THE ADVANCED PRACTICE NURSE

Kathy J. Morrison, MSN, RN, SCRN, FAHA

Diane McLaughlin, DNP, AGACNP-BC, CCRN, FCCM, FNCS

SPRINGER PUBLISHING

Springer Publishing Company, LLC
www.springerpub.com
http://connect.springerpub.com

Acquisitions Editor: John Zaphyr
Compositor: Transforma

ISBN: 978-0-8261-7603-5
ebook ISBN: 978-0-8261-7604-2
DOI: 10.1891/9780826176042

Printed by BnT

The author and the publisher of this Work have made every effort to use sources believed to be reliable to provide information that is accurate and compatible with the standards generally accepted at the time of publication. Because medical science is continually advancing, our knowledge base continues to expand. Therefore, as new information becomes available, changes in procedures become necessary. We recommend that the reader always consult current research and specific institutional policies before performing any clinical procedure or delivering any medication. The author and publisher shall not be liable for any special, consequential, or exemplary damages resulting, in whole or in part, from the readers' use of, or reliance on, the information contained in this book. The publisher has no responsibility for the persistence or accuracy of URLs for external or third-party internet websites referred to in this publication and does not guarantee that any content on such websites is, or will remain, accurate or appropriate.

Library of Congress Cataloging-in-Publication Data

Names: Morrison, Kathy (Nurse), author. | McLaughlin, Diane (Diane C.), 1977- author.
Title: Fast facts about stroke care for the advanced practice nurse / Kathy J. Morrison and Diane McLaughlin.
Other titles: Fast facts (Springer Publishing Company)
Description: First Springer Publishing edition. | New York, NY : Springer Publishing Company, [2024] | Series: Fast facts | Includes bibliographical references and index.
Identifiers: LCCN 2023020136 | ISBN 9780826176035 (paperback) | ISBN 9780826176042 (ebook)
Subjects: MESH: Stroke--nursing | Stroke--therapy | Advanced Practice Nursing
Classification: LCC RC388.5 | NLM WY 160.5 | DDC 616.8/10231--dc23/eng/20230703
LC record available at https://lccn.loc.gov/2023020136

Contact sales@springerpub.com to receive discount rates on bulk purchases.

***Publisher's Note:* New and used products purchased from third-party sellers are not guaranteed for quality, authenticity, or access to any included digital components.**

Printed in the United States of America.

I dedicate this book to Lynne Hundley, one of the most passionate advanced practice stroke nurses the world was graced to have... although for far too short a time.

—Kathy

This book is dedicated to my closest friends that continue to encourage me to chase my dreams.

—Diane

CONTENTS

CONTRIBUTORS

Brittney Bradshaw, MSN, APRN-CNP, ACNPC-AG Department of Neurology-Neurovascular, The Ohio State University Wexner Medical Center, Columbus, Ohio

Kristin Chapman, MSN, AGACNP-BC Baptist Medical Center/Lyerly Neurosurgery, Jacksonville, Florida

Erin Conahan, MSN, RN, ACNS-BC, CNRN, SCRN, PHRN Lehigh Valley Health Network, Stroke Program, Allentown, Pennsylvania

Noah Grose, MSN, APRN-CNP Department of Neurology-Neurovascular, The Ohio State University Wexner Medical Center, Columbus, Ohio

Kimberly Ichrist, DNP, AG-ACNP, CCRN The Ohio State University Wexner Medical Center, Columbus, Ohio

Martina M. Kittle, MSN, AGACNP-BC, SCRN, CNRN The Ohio State University Wexner Medical Center, Columbus, Ohio

Elizabeth J. Legros, PharmD OhioHealth Riverside, Columbus, Ohio

Justin Lowe, PA-C, ANVP Stroke Team Neurology APP, Penn State Health Milton S. Hershey Medical Center, Hershey, Pennsylvania

Jean Dougherty Luciano, MSN, RN, CNRN, SCRN, CRNP Senior Manager, Quality, Stroke & Afib, American Heart Association, Drexel Hill, Pennsylvania

Claranne Mathiesen, MSN, RN, CNRN, SCRN Neuroscience Administrator, Lehigh Valley Health Network, Allentown, Pennsylvania

Catherine Mielke, MS, APRN, CNS Nursing Education Specialist, Department of Nursing Professional Development, Mayo Clinic Florida, Jacksonville, Florida

Karen Pratt, MSN, APRN, NP-C, CCRN Nursing Education Specialist, Department of Nursing Professional Development, Mayo Clinic Florida, Jacksonville, Florida

Tina Resser, MSN, ACNP-BC, FNP-BC, CNRN Cleveland Clinic, Department of Neurosurgery, Cleveland, Ohio

Alicia Richardson, MSN, RN, ACCNS-AG, ANVP, ASC Stroke Systems Director, Penn State Health, Instructor Neurosurgery, Penn State Health Milton S. Hershey Medical Center, Hershey, Pennsylvania

Emily Rogers, DNP, APRN, AGACNP-BC, CCRN Mayo Clinic Florida, Department of Critical Care Medicine, Jacksonville, Florida

Keaton S. Smetana, PharmD, MBA, BCCCP Clinical Pharmacy Manager, OhioHealth Riverside, Columbus, Ohio

Daniel Wadden, MSN, AGACNP-BC Cleveland Clinic, Cleveland, Ohio

Randheer Yadav, DNP, APRN-CNP The Ohio State University Wexner Medical Center, Columbus, Ohio

Kaylie Yost, MSN, RN Nursing Education Specialist, Department of Nursing Professional Development, Mayo Clinic Florida, Jacksonville, Florida

PREFACE

The evolution of stroke care over the past 25 years has driven a remarkable growth in responsibility and opportunity for healthcare professionals. As research evidence led to practice standards and stroke center certification, nurses recognized that a specialty was being born. As a result, the number of stroke nursing certifications continues to grow, as does the number of nurses attaining specialized stroke certification. Over the past 5 to 10 years, it has become apparent that the same phenomenon is occurring at the advanced practice provider (APP) level of care.

Nurse practitioners, clinical nurse specialists, physician's assistants, staff/provider educators, clinical pharmacists, therapists, and other advanced healthcare professionals have long been critical members of any healthcare team, and now they have taken on stroke provider responsibilities, both inpatient and outpatient. With the success of previous *Fast Facts* stroke care books, it became clear that this group of APPs would benefit from a similar resource.

This *Fast Facts* book has been designed to provide comprehensive, concise, advanced stroke care information across the continuum of care. We gathered healthcare experts from across the country to contribute chapters in line with their own stroke subspecialty. The intent is for APPs working in critical care units, stroke units, rehabilitation units, emergency departments, interventional suites, operating rooms, outpatient clinics, primary care offices, and pharmacies, along with those who educate them, to find this book valuable.

There are now stroke/vascular certifications for advanced level providers that this book would help to prepare candidates pursuing those certifications. Organizations that oversee comprehensive stroke certification have recognized the valuable role of APPs as part of the overall stroke care team, by requiring such in their standards.

Stroke research continues to expand across all aspects of care, treatment, and therapy providing a steady stream of new evidence that continues to improve the outcomes of our stroke patients. The opportunities for APPs in this challenging and evidence-rich population are endless.

If you have any comments or suggestions for this book, or want to contact me, please do so at kmorrison98@gmail.com.

Kathy J. Morrison

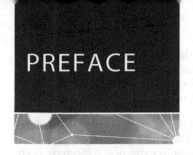

During my time at the bedside, I have seen the evolution of stroke care first-hand. Ironically, once the easiest patients to take care of—as there was nothing to do—stroke patients now have the chance for meaningful recovery thanks to advances in both medical management and interventions, including thrombolysis and thrombectomy.

One of my favorite statistics to recite is that neurology is every year voted the most difficult specialty by medical students. There continues to be a gap in the number of neurologists needed and the amount in existence. APPs have been identified as crucial to help bridge this gap. Specialty education is needed to help facilitate this, and this book can help you get started. Even with decades in this field, I learned new things just editing these chapters. I highly urge anyone working with stroke patients to read this book, keep it handy, and share it with others in the field. It has been my pleasure to work on this and see care of the stroke patient through discovery to recovery.

If you have any comments or suggestions for this book, or want to contact me, please do so at mclaughlin.diane@mayo.edu.

Diane McLaughlin

ACKNOWLEDGMENTS

We would like to acknowledge the following people for their contributions: Rachel Landes for introducing Kathy and Diane in order to work on this book together. Joe Morita for continuing to support our vision for this project over the course of years. John Zaphyr for picking up this project 2 years in and shepherding it home. Springer Publishing for believing in our book enough to publish it. Nicholas McLaughlin for the outstanding illustrations in Chapter 3. Our contributing authors who add years of knowledge and expertise and were willing to share it with the world. All of our patients who continue to inspire us to make a difference.

1

SECTION I: INTRODUCTION

The Role of the Advanced Practice Provider in Stroke Care

Diane McLaughlin and Kristin Chapman

Stroke is one of the most common causes of mortality and disability in the world. Despite advances leading to decreased stroke-related mortality, the incidence of stroke continues to rise. Additionally, stroke survivors are at risk for recurrent ischemic stroke, with this occurring in 5% to 15% of patients. Research has shown that modifiable risk factors (hypertension, smoking, obesity, diet, and physical activity) account for most strokes. Lifestyle modification and appropriate medication management are crucial in secondary stroke prevention.

In the United States, there is a current shortage of neurologists, with the demand for additional neurologists expected to outpace the supply. By 2025, the deficit is anticipated to reach nearly 20%. Many organizations have recognized the use of advanced practice providers (APPs) to help bridge the gap. The American Academy of Neurology (2020) released a statement supporting the use of APPs to support access to neurologic care in 2015 and updated the statement in 2020 to clarify the use of APPs within a physician-led multidisciplinary team, while supporting the use of all members to practice at the full extent of their licensure and training (Dall et al., 2013). This chapter outlines the expansion of the APP role in stroke care.

INPATIENT ROLES

Code Strokes

A code stroke is called whenever a patient has signs and symptoms that may be due to stroke. Facial asymmetry, focal motor weakness, slurred speech or aphasia, and sensory changes are some symptoms for which code strokes may be called. APPs are often utilized to perform rapid assessment and evaluation of patients presenting with suspected stroke. They aid in expeditiously identifying patients eligible for intravenous thrombolytic therapy and/or endovascular intervention.

Role of the Advanced Practice Provider in Code Strokes

- Act as first responders.
- Obtain relevant history from the patient or their families—key data such as last known well (LWK) or time of onset of stroke symptoms, and review of medications, particularly anticoagulants.
- Perform rapid National Institutes of Health Stroke Scale (NIHSS) assessment.
- Expedite neuroimaging and interpretation of imaging in real time.
- Review contraindications for tissue plasminogen activator (tPA).
- Facilitate rapid administration of tPA when applicable.
- Coordinate rapid transfer to the interventional radiology (IR)/endovascular suite when indicated for mechanical thrombectomy.
- Facilitate triage of patients to the appropriate hospital unit (ICU/stroke unit, etc.).

The Code Stroke APP can be under departments of stroke neurology, neurosurgery, critical care, ED, or as a dedicated rapid responder to medical emergencies. APP responders allow for parallel workflow among the stroke neurologist, ED nurses and physicians, as well as other primary and consulting groups. Data comparing stroke codes run by highly trained, specialized APPs demonstrated faster door-to-needle (DTN) times and door-to-groin times in the APP group in comparison with medical residents, with a more accurate final diagnosis in the form of stroke (Grose et al., 2021).

Stroke Neurology

APPs employed in stroke neurology or generalized neurology often involve the immediate care and follow-up care for patients admitted with stroke or transient ischemic attack (TIA). These APPs may have inpatient and outpatient roles.

Role of the Stroke Neurology Advanced Practice Provider

- Attend and actively participate in acute code stroke activations.
- Provide continuity of care for these patients by co-managing, supporting, and supplementing acute stroke care provided by the stroke neurologist by virtue of daily rounding on stroke inpatients.
- Ensure that stroke metrics are met in the process as established by the American Heart Association (AHA) "Get With the Guidelines."
  - Swallow evaluation
  - Appropriately and timely follow-up of neuroimaging
  - Discharge planning including rehabilitation facility referral and review of most appropriate medications for secondary stroke prevention and setting up follow-up clinical appointments after discharge

Neurovascular/Neurosurgery/Neurointervention

Neurovascular, neurosurgery, or neurointervention APPs take an active role in surveillance of patients at high risk for requiring intervention and of patients requiring urgent and definitive treatment. These APPs also are utilized to provide both inpatient and outpatient follow-up for stroke patients that had intervention performed or remain at risk for possible future intervention. They often scrub into procedures and are involved with post-procedural monitoring.

Role of the Neurovascular Advanced Practice Provider

- Assess patients potentially requiring intervention.
- Coordinate with IR and assemble the team.
- Transporti stroke patients to the thrombectomy suite.
- Facilitate a reduction in door-to-groin puncture times by obtaining arterial vascular access to expedite clot retrieval.
- Remove sheath.
- Assess serial surgical site.
- Provide post-procedural care and follow-up.

Critical Care/Neurocritical Care

Critical care APPs manage patients that are acutely ill either by hemodynamic criteria (requiring titration of continuous infusions, such as vasopressors, antihypertensives), airway criteria (requiring intervention or high risk for imminent deterioration requiring intervention), or neurologic criteria (may develop cerebral edema, hemorrhage expansion or transformation, or hydrocephalus). These APPs may be staff of a general critical care department, neurology department, or neurosurgery department.

Role of the Critical Care Advanced Practice Provider

- Participate directly in the code stroke process.
  - Initial patient evaluation
  - Administration of IV thrombolytic therapy
- Monitor the patient for complications of stroke.
- Provide blood pressure management.
  - Acute lowering
  - Blood pressure augmentation for patients with perfusion dependent examination
- Administer airway management.
- Provide cerebral edema management.
- Monitor for acute herniation syndrome and provide acute management for osmotherapy, short-term hyperventilation, and potentially coordinating surgical management.
- Provide procedural management: arterial lines, central lines, intubation, bronchoscopy, extraventricular drain (EVD) placement.
- Coordinate disposition plan.
- Administer stroke workup.

FAST FACTS

A single-center retrospective cohort study at Queen's Medical Center in Honolulu from 2009 to 2014 showed that the median DTN time was reduced from 53 minutes to 45 minutes and the median imaging-to-needle (ITN) time was reduced from 36 minutes to 21 minutes after the introduction of a 24/7 acute care nurse practitioner (ACNP) first responder coverage for a hospital stroke code team (Moran et al., 2016).

Stroke Coordinator/Nurse Educator

APPs also serve in the vital role of stroke coordinator or stroke navigator by

- Providing inpatient stroke education, including nursing staff education regarding IV thrombolytic mixing/administration, and performing a focused neurologic exam.
- Ensuring best practices and stroke quality measures are met.
- Reviewing all thrombolytic and thrombectomy cases for delays and complications.
- Performing thorough chart audits.
- Ensuring quality improvement and compliance with Joint Commission requirements for certification and recertification.
- APPs also serve in the role of nurse educators, either as a dedicated position or a supplementary role to their primary clinical responsibilities.

There is clear evidence that stroke coordinators are associated with reduced stay length and improved delivery of evidence-based care in hospitals with a stroke unit (Purvis et al., 2018; Rattray et al., 2017).

OUTPATIENT ROLES

Stroke Follow-Up

APPs play a large role in providing follow-up care for stroke outpatients. Outpatient care can be administered in the clinic, through home visits, or via telemedicine.

Patient Teaching

- Controlling hypertension, hyperlipidemia, diabetes
- Chronic anticoagulation for atrial fibrillation—reinitiation, management, patient teaching
- Smoking cessation
- Diet, physical activity

Depression Screening

- Depression is common after stroke, and early intervention will ensure continuation of therapies and social interaction.

Medication Compliance

- Early discontinuation of statin therapy (3–6 months) is associated with high risk of recurrent stroke.
- There is increased risk of stroke when aspirin is stopped.
- A nurse practitioner (NP)-led transitional stroke clinic developed at Wake Forest Medical Center reduced readmission rates at 30 days by about 50% (Condon et al., 2016).
- Identify and address barriers to taking medications as prescribed.

Plan of Care Compliance

- Monitor consistency of physical, occupational, and speech therapy appointments.
- Identify and address barriers to keeping therapy or follow-up appointments.

Caregiver Support

- Monitor caregiver during follow-up interaction for signs of stress, depression, and self-care neglect.
- Make recommendations for social support services such as a stroke support group or outpatient social work consult.

FAST FACTS

In their study of the impact of APRNs on a stroke follow-up clinic, Mitchell's group demonstrated that by utilizing these APRNs, the time to clinic follow-up was reduced from 116.9 days to 33.6 days and unplanned readmissions within 30 days declined from 11.5% to 9.9% (Mitchell et al., 2022).

MOBILE STROKE

Mobile stroke units equipped with CT capabilities are becoming more commonplace with various staffing models. One study compared APP to MD within mobile stroke units and found that diagnosis agreement was 100% for strokes and 98% for stroke mimics. Additionally, intracerebral hemorrhage (ICH) identification/treatment agreement was 100%; tPA administration was 98%, with APPs more likely to be slightly more conservative. The use of APPs in this independent role was proven to be noninferior to an appropriately qualified physician and hence safe and feasible (Alexandrov et al., 2017).

PRIMARY CARE

APPs in the primary care provider (PCP) role who are familiar with primary prevention guidelines are in the perfect position to ensure proper risk factor control, giving their patient the best chance of stroke prevention. They are also critically important in stroke follow-up for secondary prevention as described earlier.

STROKE RESEARCH

APPs in the role of Stroke Research Coordinators enroll and follow up with study participants. They are also principal investigators (PIs) on a growing number of nurse-driven studies.

SUMMARY

The opportunities for APPs to participate in stroke care continue to increase. They contribute in a variety of settings and have greatly enhanced the ability to meet stroke patients' needs, particularly in the setting of limited neurologists nationwide. All evidence shows that APPs improve stroke care in any role that has been studied. Further details of care are discussed in each setting throughout the course of this book.

References

Alexandrov, A. W., Dusenbury, W., Swatzell, V., Rike, J., Bouche, A., Crisp, I., Jestice, M., Fletcher, J., Crockett, M., Ware, T., Stacks, W., Barber, I., McDevitt, P., McDaniel, S., Mathenia, T., Orr, J., McKendry, C., Novak, T., Bey, S., … & Alexandrov, A. V. (2017). Born to run: Advanced practice provider-led mobile stroke unit care measures up to vascular neurologists' diagnoses and management. *Stroke, 48*, ANS6. https://doi.org/10.1161/str.48.suppl_1.ns6

American Academy of Neurology. (2020). *Position statement: Neurology advanced practice providers.* https://www.aan.com/siteassets/home-page/policy-and-guidelines/policy/position-statements/neurology-advanced-practice-providers/21-app-position-statement.pdf

Condon, C., Lycan, S., Duncan, P., & Bushnell, C. (2016). Reducing readmissions after stroke with a structured nurse practitioner/registered nurse transitional stroke program. *Stroke, 47,* 1599–1604. https://doi.org/10.1161/STROKEAHA.115.012524

Dall, T. M., Storm, M. V., Chakrabarti, R., Drogan, O., Keran, C. M., Donofrio, P. D., Henderson, V. W., Kaminski, H. J., Stevens, J. C., & Vidic, T. R. (2013). Supply and demand analysis of the current and future US neurology workforce. *Neurology, 81*(5), 470–478. https://doi.org/10.1212/WNL.0b013e318294b1cf

Grose, N., Forrest, C., Heaton, S., & Lee, V. (2021). Advanced practice provider-based acute stroke protocol performs well compared to a resident-based protocol. *Stroke, 52*, AP32. https://doi.org/10.1161/str.52.suppl_1.P32

Mitchell, M., Reynolds, S., Mower-Wade, D., Raser-Schramm, J., & Granger, B. (2022). Implementation of an advanced practice registered nurse-led clinic to improve follow-up care for post-ischemic stroke patients. *Journal of Neuroscience Nursing, 54*(5), 193–198. https://doi.org/10.1097/JNN.0000000000000670

Moran, J. L., Nakagawa, K., Asai, S. M., & Koenig, M. A. (2016). 24/7 neurocritical care nurse practitioner coverage reduced door-to-needle time in stroke patients treated with tissue plasminogen activator. *Journal of Stroke and Cerebrovascular Diseases, 25*, 1148–1152.

Purvis, T., Kilkenney, M. F., Middleton, S., & Cadilhac, D. A. (2018). Influence of stroke coordinators on delivery of acute stroke care and hospital outcomes: An observational study. *International Journal of Stroke, 13*, 585–591. https://doi.org/10.1177/1747493017741382

Rattray, N. A., Damush, T. M., Luckhurst, C., Bauer-Martinez, C. J., Homoya, B. J., & Miech, E. J. (2017). Prime movers: Advanced practice professionals in the role of stroke coordinator. *Journal of the American Association of Nurse Practitioners, 29*, 392–402. https://doi.org/10.1002/2327-6924.12462

Stroke Care Evolution

Kathy J. Morrison

While the evolution of stroke care must begin with its first recognition in 400 BCE, it is worthwhile to understand how it evolved into the major healthcare topic that it is today; and it's only been fairly recently—the 20th century—that stroke care evolved beyond supportive and rehabilitative care.

- ***400 BCE: Hippocrates described episodes of convulsions and paralysis, typically on the opposite side of the injury, along with episodes of impaired speech as apoplexy.***
- ***1689: William Cole used the term* stroke *for the first time in reference to a health condition.***
- ***1890: This was the first time that* stroke *appeared in nursing texts regarding supportive care—and only if the patient survived the stroke and the many secondary injuries that often accompanied stroke (Nilsen, 2010).***

Prior to the 20th century, the three leading causes of death were pneumonia, tuberculosis (TB), and diarrhea/enteritis. The medical professionals were focused on treating infectious diseases to keep people alive rather than thinking about disease prevention. They made significant strides during the 19th century that set up the 20th century scientific and medical community to continue to improve public health.

19TH-CENTURY DEVELOPMENTS

- **1854:** discovery of microorganisms that caused many infectious diseases like cholera and TB
- **1855:** improved sanitation systems and hygiene standards
- **1897:** chlorination of drinking water (Department of Health and Human Services, 1999a)

During the first half of the 20th century, many diseases were eradicated, changing the cause of death statistics. The three leading causes of death became heart disease, cancer, and stroke. The medical community realized a vastly different challenge with heart disease and stroke, together accounting for 40% of all deaths (Department of Health and Human Services, 1999b).

20TH-CENTURY DEVELOPMENTS: 1900 TO 1950

- **1918 to 1920:** pasteurization of milk and refrigeration
- **1928 to 1948:** penicillin, and streptomycin for TB
- **1930 to 1950:** public education on handwashing and food safety provided by local health departments

The second half of the 20th century was marked by myriad research into heart disease and stroke—causes, treatments, risk factors, and so forth—that has led to remarkable improvements in heart disease and stroke mortality. Heart disease deaths dropped by 60% and stroke deaths dropped by 70%.

20TH-CENTURY DEVELOPMENTS: 1951 TO 1999

- **1970:** The World Health Organization (WHO) defined stroke as "rapidly developing clinical signs of focal or global disturbance of cerebral function, lasting more than 24 hours or leading to death, with no apparent cause other than that of vascular origin" (Sacco et al., 2013).
- **1996:** The first emergency treatment for stroke was approved by the Food and Drug Administration (FDA)—tissue plasminogen activator (tPA), or alteplase.
- **2000:** Brain Attack Coalition's *Recommendations for the Establishment of Primary Stroke Centers* was published.
- **2015:** Mechanical clot retrieval became the standard of care for large vessel occlusion (LVO) strokes.

The 21st century has already seen countless guidelines and recommendations that resulted from 20th-century research—and that research continues. We are now equipped with real evidence proving that focused care and timely treatments absolutely do impact outcomes … not just on the emergency side, but with post-acute care as well. This is an exciting time for healthcare professionals involved in stroke care at all levels, and it is no wonder that the role of the advanced practice provider (APP) has become so significant in stroke care.

STROKE-SPECIFIC PROFESSIONAL CERTIFICATION PROGRAMS

The specialty of stroke care has impacted not only nursing but also prehospital and ED providers, physician assistants (PAs), stroke coordinators, educators for nurses, and APPs. The list of stroke-specific certification programs will only grow throughout the 21st century as evidence shows that certification in stroke care results in a higher level of knowledge and care, as well as improved outcomes for our patients.

- **ASLS**: Acute Stroke Life Support is a certification program for prehospital and emergency healthcare professionals established in 1998 by the Gordon Center, University of Miami.
- **NVRN**: Neurovascular Registered Nurse was established in 2007 by the Association of Neurovascular Clinicians (ANVC).

- **ANVP**: Advanced Neurovascular Provider was established in 2007 by the ANVC.
- **NET SMART**: Neurovascular Education and Training in Stroke Management and Acute Reperfusion Therapy, a post-graduate fellowship training program for nurses and APPs, was established by Anne Alexandrov in 2007.
- **SCRN**: Stroke Certified Registered Nurse was established in 2012 by the American Board of Neuroscience Nursing (ABNN).
- **CSRS**: Certified Stroke Rehabilitation Specialist was established in 2012 by Neurorecovery Unlimited.
- **ASC-BC**: Advanced Stroke Coordinator-Board Certified was established in 2019 by the ANVC.

STROKE-RELATED PROFESSIONAL CERTIFICATION PROGRAMS

Particularly in the prehospital realm, professional certifications that enhance stroke care by emergency medical technicians (EMTs), paramedics, nurses, and APPs have become available and are becoming more numerous.

- **ENLS**: Emergency Neurologic Life Support was established in 2010 by the Neurocritical Care Society
- **PHRN**: Prehospital Registered Nurse was established in the early 2000s; availability and recognition varies by state

STROKE-SPECIFIC HOSPITAL CERTIFICATION PROGRAMS

Just as with professional certification programs, the number of organizations with stroke certification has grown tremendously in the 21st century. Most states require their prehospital personnel to be able to identify suspected stroke symptoms, identify the likelihood of an LVO, and then take the patient to the appropriate stroke center.

In 2022, there were 2,448 certified stroke centers: 297 comprehensive stroke centers (CSCs), 14 thrombectomy-capable stroke centers (TSCs), 1,459 primary stroke centers (PSCs), and 678 acute stroke-ready hospitals (ASRHs; Boggs et al., 2022). This represents a 64% increase from 2009, when there were 876 certified stroke centers, mostly PSCs, as this was the first level to be designated in 2003, followed by CSC in 2012, ASRH in 2015, and TSC in 2018.

STROKE CENTER CAPABILITIES

Acute Stroke-Ready Hospital

- Rapid evaluation of acute stroke and administration of IV thrombolytic; neurologic evaluation is often provided via telemedicine and teleradiology; transfer of intervention candidates to a CSC or TSC, complex cases to a CSC, with other stroke patients going to a PSC.

Primary Stroke Center

- Rapid evaluation of acute stroke and administration of IV thrombolytic; admitting and treating most stroke patients, with transfer agreement for sending intervention candidates and complex cases to a CSC; compliance with stroke (STK) measures

Thrombectomy-Capable Stroke Center

- Same as PSC, but with additional capability of performing emergent mechanical clot retrieval; requirement for minimum of 12 thrombectomies/provider annually; compliance with STK measures and five of the comprehensive stroke (CSTK) measures

Comprehensive Stroke Center

- Treats the most complex stroke patients, including hemorrhagic strokes; mechanical clot retrieval for ischemic strokes; research protocols in various aspects of stroke care; dedicated neuro intensive care unit; compliance with STK and CSTK measures

Stroke Rehabilitation Certification

- Stroke-certified therapists and stroke oversight team that provides evidence of compliance with best practice standards, use of clinical practice guidelines, quality metrics and performance improvement initiatives.

FAST FACTS

There is a common misconception that The Joint Commission (TJC) was responsible for coming up with the standards for PSCs, probably because they were the first to offer certification, coupled with their reputation as an authority on hospital accreditation. However, it was The Brain Attack Coalition that established these standards in their publication, "Recommendations for the Establishment of Primary Stroke Centers" (Albers et al., 2000).

ORGANIZATIONS THAT PROVIDE STROKE CENTER CERTIFICATION

The Joint Commission

- Founded in 1951 with the mission of improving healthcare (www.joint commission.org/about_us/history.aspx)
- Oldest and largest accrediting and standards-setting organization in healthcare
- First organization to establish a program for PSC certification in 2003 through its Disease-Specific Care Division; also has ASRH, TSC, and CSC certification programs; certification valid for 2 years
- Only organization providing Stroke Rehabilitation certification

Healthcare Facilities Accreditation Program

- Created in 1945 for the purpose of review of osteopathic hospitals (www.hfap.org/CertificationPrograms/certificationProcess.aspx)
- Broadened its scope to all hospitals in 1965
- Since 2008 has provided certification; also provides Acute Stroke-Ready, Thrombectomy-Capable, and CSC certifications
- Certification valid for 3 years

Det Norse Veritas

- Founded in Norway; Det Norse Veritas established an American presence in 1897 with an initial focus on risk-management consulting for the maritime industry (www.dnvgl.us/assurance/healthcare/stroke-certs.html)
- Healthcare division approved by Centers for Medicare & Medicaid Services (CMS) in 2007 as an accrediting organization
- Certification valid for 3 years; also provides Acute Stroke-Ready, Thrombectomy-Capable, and CSC certifications

Center for Improvement in Healthcare Quality

- Founded in 1999 in McKinney, Texas (www.cihq.org/)
- Disease-specific certification, of which stroke is a part, founded in 2019
- Certification valid for 3 years; also provides Acute Stroke Ready, Thrombectomy-Capable, and CSC certifications

STROKE MEASURES

The original 10 stroke performance measures were developed in November 2004 by the blood alcohol concentration (BAC), in collaboration with the American Heart Association/American Stroke Association (AHA/ASA). The purpose was to support PSC certification. These 10 measures were based on research evidence of processes that resulted in improved outcomes for stroke patients. Organizations pursuing PSC certification and recertification had to demonstrate compliance with—or performance improvement strategies toward—all 10 of the measures.

From 2008 to 2015, eight of the 10 stroke performance measures were endorsed by the National Quality Forum (NQF) as core measures and were aligned with the CMS's measures. The two that were not endorsed were dysphagia screening and tobacco-cessation counseling. Dysphagia screening was not endorsed due to the lack of a valid, reliable, standardized screening tool or process supported by research (Hickey & Livesay, 2015), although it is recognized as an important aspect of prevention of aspiration pneumonia. Smoking cessation was not endorsed as it was deemed to have already been met by organizational initiatives and through documentation of teaching or counseling provided.

The Stroke Core Measures were retired as Core Measures on December 31, 2015, by the CMS, but continue to be required for performance measure reporting for stroke center certification, thus are performance measures. It is not uncommon for healthcare professionals to continue to refer to them as Core Measures, although technically incorrect.

With the growth of additional stroke center certification levels, there have come along additional stroke measures. Tables 2.1, 2.2, 2.3, and 2.4, and Figure 2.1 provide an overview of the current measures for which compliance is required for stroke center certification.

TABLE 2.1

Stroke Measures

STK-1	VTE Prophylaxis
STK-2	Discharged on Antithrombotic Therapy
STK-3	Anticoagulation Therapy for Atrial Fibrillation/Flutter
STK-4	Thrombolytic Therapy
STK-5	Antithrombotic Therapy by End of Hospital Day 2
STK-6	Discharged on Statin Medication
STK-8	Stroke Education
STK-10	Assessed for Rehabilitation

STK, stroke; VTE, venous thromboembolism.

TABLE 2.2

Stroke Outpatient Measures for EDs in Non-Comprehensive Stroke Centers

STK-OP-1	Door to Transfer to Another Hospital
STK-OP-1a	Overall Rate
STK-OP-1b	Hemorrhagic Stroke
STK-OP-1d	Ischemic Stroke; No IV Alteplase Prior to Transfer, LVO and MER Eligible
STK-OP-1e	Ischemic Stroke; No IV Alteplase Prior to Transfer, LVO and NOT MER Eligible
STK-OP-1f	Ischemic Stroke; No IV Alteplase Prior to Transfer, No LVO
STK-OP-1g	Ischemic Stroke; IV Alteplase Prior to Transfer, LVO and MER Eligible
STK-OP-1h	Ischemic Stroke; IV Alteplase Prior to Transfer, LVO and NOT MER Eligible
STK-OP-1i	Ischemic Stroke; IV Alteplase Prior to Transfer, No LVO

LVO, large vessel occlusion; MER, mechanical thrombectomy; OP, outpatient; STK, stroke.

TABLE 2.3

Outpatient Stroke

OP-23	Head CT or MRI Scan Results for Acute Ischemic Stroke or Hemorrhagic Stroke Patients Who Received Head CT or MRI Scan Interpretation Within 45 Minutes of ED Arrival

OP, outpatient; STK, stroke.

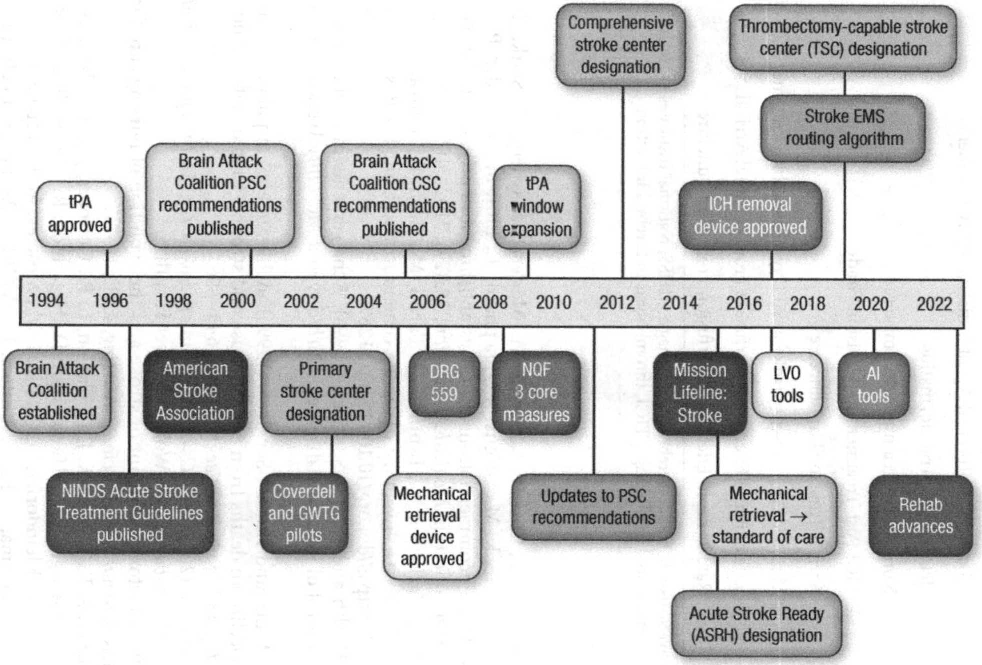

Figure 2.1 Acute stroke milestones.

AI, artificial intelligence; CSC, comprehensive stroke center; DRG, diagnosis-related group; EMS, emergency medical services; GWTG, Get With the Guidelines; ICH, intracerebral hemorrhage; LVO, large-vessel occlusion; NINDS, National Institute of Neurological Disorders and Stroke; NQF, National Quality Forum; PSC, primary stroke center; TJC, The Joint Commission; tPA, tissue plasminogen activator.

TABLE 2.4

Comprehensive Stroke Measures

CSTK-01	NIHSS Performed for Ischemic Stroke Patients
CSTK-03	Severity Measurement Performed for SAH and ICH Patients
CSTK-04	Procoagulant Reversal Agent Initiation for ICH Patients
CSTK-05	Hemorrhagic Transformation
CSTK-06	Nimodipine Treatment Administered
CSTK-08	TICI Post-Treatment Reperfusion Grade
CSTK-09	Arrival Time to Skin Puncture
CSTK-10	Modified Rankin Score (mRS at 90 Days: Favorable Outcome)
CSTK-11	Rate of Rapid Effective Reperfusion From Hospital Arrival
CSTK-12	Rate of Rapid Effective Reperfusion From Skin Puncture

CSTK, comprehensive stroke; ICH, intracerebral hemorrhage; NIHSS, National Institutes of Health Stroke Scale; SAH, subarachnoid hemorrhage; TICI, thrombolysis in cerebral infarction.

References

Albers, M., Hademenos, G., Latchaw, R., Jagoda, A., Marler, J., Mayberg, M., Starke, R. D., Todd, H. W., Viste, K. M., Girgus, M., Shephard, T., Emr, M., Shwayder, P., & Walker, M. (2000). Recommendations for the establishment of primary stroke centers. *Journal of the American Medical Association*, *283*(23), 3102–3109.

Boggs, K., Vogel, B., Zachrison, K., Espinola, J., Faridi, M., Cash, R., Sullivan, A., & Camargo, C. (2022). An inventory of stroke centers in the United States. *JACEP Open*, *3*, e12673. https://doi.org/10.1002/emp2.12673

Department of Health and Human Services. (1999a). Achievements in public health, 1900–1999: Control of infectious diseases. *Morbidity and Mortality Weekly*, *48*(29), 621–629.

Department of Health and Human Services. (1999b). Achievements in public health, 1900–1999: Decline in deaths from heart disease and stroke—United States, 1900–1999. *Morbidity and Mortality Weekly*, *48*(30), 649–656.

Hickey, J., & Livesay, S. (2015). *The C = continuum of stroke care: An interprofessional approach to evidence-based care*. Wolters Kluwer Health.

Nilsen, M. (2010). A historical account of stroke and the evolution of nursing care for stroke patients. *Journal of Neuroscience Nursing*, *42*(1), 19–27.

Sacco, R. L., Kasner, S. E., Broderick, J. P., Caplan, L. R., Connors, J. J., Culebras, A., Elkind, M. S. V., George, M. G., Hamdan, A. D., Higashida, R. T., Hoh, B. L., Scott Janis, L., Kase, C. S., Kleindorfer, D. O., Lee, J.-M., Moseley, M. E., Peterson, E. D., Turan, T. N., Valderrama, A. L., … Vinters, H. V. (2013). An updated definition of stroke for the 21st century: A statement for healthcare professionals from the American Heart Association/American Stroke Association. *Stroke*, *44*, 2064–2089.

3

Advanced Anatomy and Physiology

Kathy J. Morrison

Illustrations Contributor: Nicholas McLaughlin

The advanced practice provider (APP) working with stroke patients must be familiar and comfortable with neurovascular anatomy and function in order to understand their patients' presentation and prognosis. Developing a plan of care, understanding discharge plan of care, and educating patients, families, and other healthcare professionals will be greatly enhanced with a solid knowledge of cerebral and cerebellar function and vascular supply patterns.

REVIEW OF BASICS

Within the skull, the brain is further protected by three meningeal layers (see Figure 3.1).

Dura Mater

- **Dura mater:** thick, fibrous connective tissue that closely lines the inside of the skull. There are two dural folds:
  - The falx separates the right and left hemispheres of the brain.
  - The tentorium separates the cerebrum from the cerebellum.
- **Arachnoid mater:** delicate fibrous membrane attached to the dura mater
  - Named for the delicate, spiderweb-like filaments that extend to the pia mater
- **Pia mater:** thin membrane that covers the surface of the brain
  - Fits the brain like a latex glove fits the hand, following the surface detail of the sulci and gyri

The brain is divided into two hemispheres, separated by the longitudinal fissure, with connection being the corpus callosum (Figure 3.2).

The outer portion of the hemispheres is the cerebral cortex, also known as gray matter. It contains sulci and gyri (grooves and folds) that increase the surface of the brain (Figure 3.2). The four lobes of the cortex are:

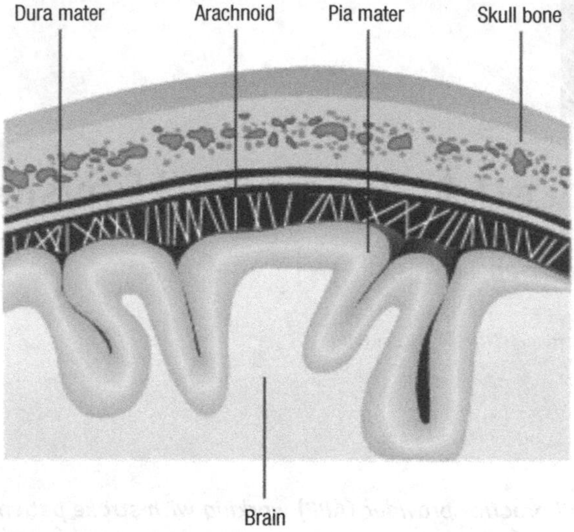

Figure 3.1 Meninges layers.

Source: Morrison, K. (2023). *Stroke nursing certification review*. Springer Publishing Company.

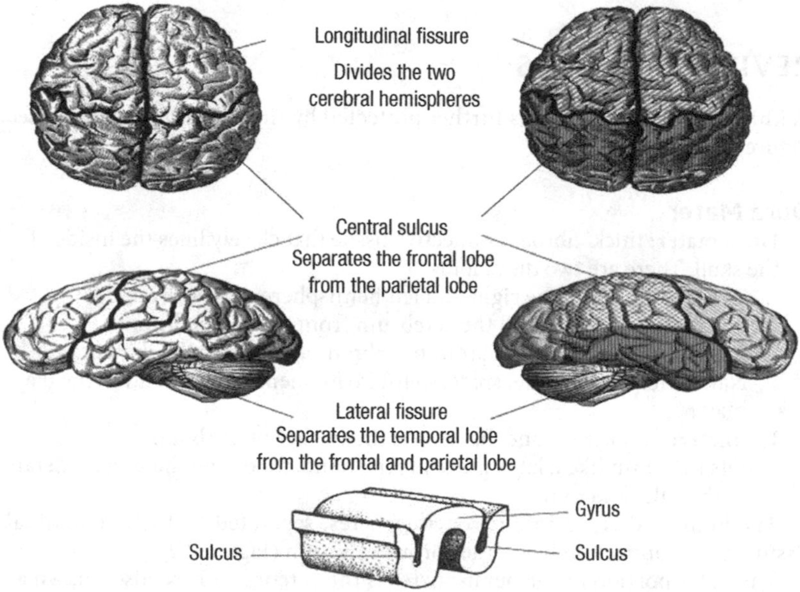

Figure 3.2 Cortical sulci/fissures and gyri.

Source: Courtesy of Nicholas McLaughlin.

- Frontal lobe
  - Anterior portion is the prefrontal lobe or prefrontal cortex; functions are planning and initiation, personality expression, and moderation of social behaviors.
  - Posterior portion is the primary motor cortex or motor strip; it is also called the precentral gyrus because it lies in front of the central sulcus.
  - Broca's area is responsible for language production, or motor speech.
- Parietal lobe
  - Anterior portion is the primary sensory cortex or sensory strip; it is also called the postcentral gyrus; function is to process sensory input.
  - Right parietal lobe function is interpretation of the position of the body in relation to its surroundings.
  - Left parietal lobe function includes the ability to understand numbers and manipulation of objects.
- Occipital lobe
  - Functions are visual spatial processing, color recognition, and motion perception
- Temporal lobe
  - Functions are hearing, memory, facial and object recognition, and receptive speech
  - Wernicke's area is located in the area of the temporal lobe called the primary auditory cortex; function is speech processing, or receptive speech

The homunculus is a diagram that depicts which parts of the body are controlled by the motor and sensory strips. The top of the motor/sensory strip controls the lower portion of the body (legs and feet), whereas the bottom of the motor/sensory strip controls the upper portion of the body (face and arms; Figure 3.3).

The fact that the motor and sensory strips are adjacent facilitates sensory motor integration. Sensory information from the body helps to inform and control the extent of motor output. For instance, touching a hot stove will produce a painful, hot sensation, and when that message is received in the sensory strip, it produces a rapid motor response to withdraw the hand from the hot stove.

FAST FACTS

The terms gray matter and white matter originated with early neuroanatomy research using slices of tissue dyed to differentiate structures for microscopic examination. The cells that make up the cortex stained easily, whereas the myelin-covered tracts of subcortical structures did not.

Subcortical Structures

Beneath the cortex is the white matter, which contains tracts of axons; this area is referred to as the subcortical space. This is a group of diverse formations, a mix of gray and white matter that provide more primitive functions than the cerebral cortex such as hunger and emotions; however, the cortex and

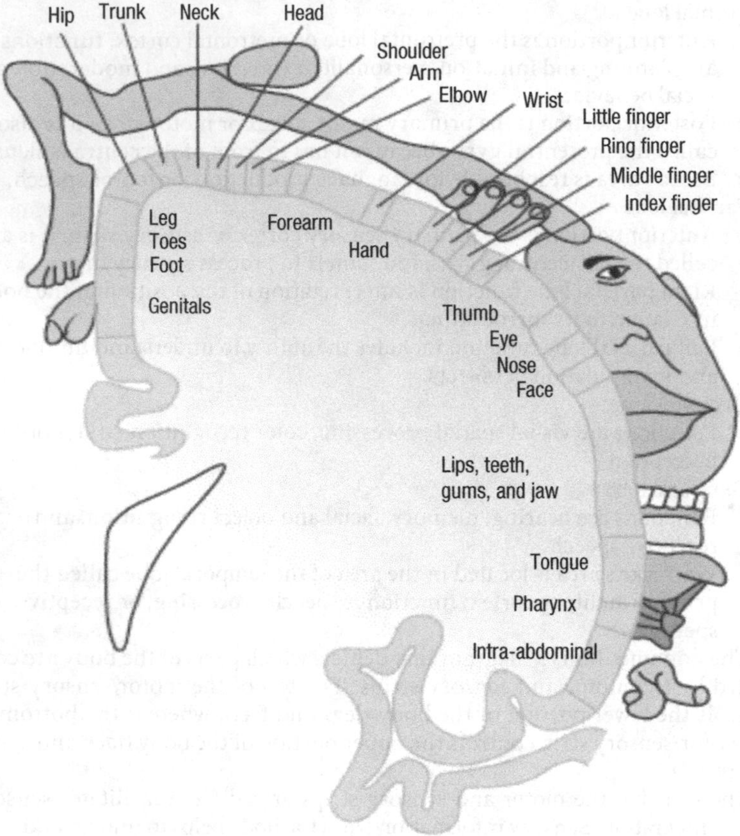

Figure 3.3 Homunculus.

Source: Morrison, K. (2023). *Stroke nursing certification review*. Springer Publishing Company.

subcortex are continually interacting and one without the other would not be feasible (Figure 3.4).

- Internal capsule
  - Allows communication between areas of the cerebral cortex and areas of the brainstem. These connections are made possible by the pathways of the internal capsule and are necessary for physical movement and perception of sensory information.
- External capsule
  - Connects the cerebral cortex to another cortical area
- Extreme capsule
  - A long association fiber pathway of white matter in the brain that provides bidirectional communication between such areas as the claustrum and the insular cortex, and the inferior frontal gyrus and the middle-posterior portion of the superior temporal gyrus

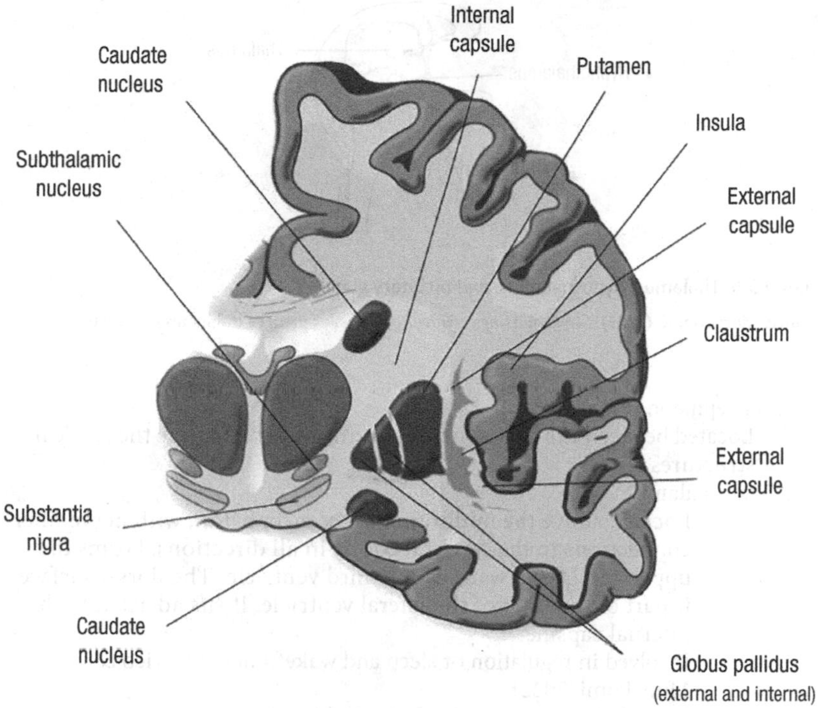

Figure 3.4 Basal ganglia/subcortical structures.

Source: Courtesy of Nicholas McLaughlin.

- Insula
  - Controls autonomic functions through the regulation of the sympathetic and parasympathetic systems. It has a role in regulating the immune system.
- Claustrum
  - Acts as a conductor for inputs from the cortical regions so these respective areas do not become unsynchronized
- Basal ganglia
  - Caudate nucleus, putamen, globus pallidus, subthalamic nucleus, and substantia nigra (SN)
  - The caudate putamen (CP) or corpus striatum is a central component of the basal ganglia, performing critical functions in the integration of information including motor control, cognition, and emotion.
  - Globus pallidus icontrols conscious and proprioceptive movements
  - Subthalamic nucleus is movement regulation along with the rest of the basal ganglia
  - SN is a part of your brain that helps control your movements.

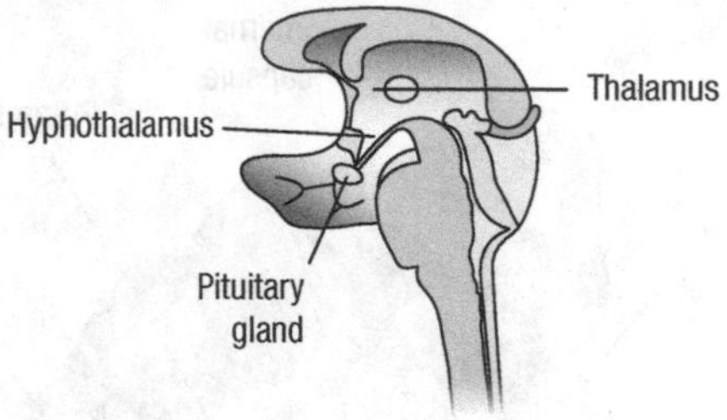

Figure 3.5 Thalamus, hypothalamus, and pituitary gland.

Source: Morrison, K. (2023). *Stroke nursing certification review*. Springer Publishing Company.

- Diencephalon (Figure 3.5)
  - Located between the hemispheres and are gray matter like the cortical structures
    - Thalamus
      - Located above the midbrain or mesencephalon, with nerve fiber connections to the cerebral cortex in all directions. Forms the upper and lateral walls of the third ventricle. The dorsal surface is part of the floor of the lateral ventricle. It sits adjacent to the internal capsule.
      - Involved in regulation of sleep and wakefulness (Torrico & Munakomi, 2022)
      - Spinothalamic tract is the pathway for pain, temperature, and crude touch. Dejerine-Roussy syndrome or thalamic pain syndrome is a rare condition following thalamic stroke. Initial presentation is the absence of sensation with tingling of the body contralateral to the affected thalamus; months later, numbness occurs, evolving into severe chronic pain.
      - Blood supplied by basilar communicating artery, posterior cerebral artery (PCA), and posterior communicating artery
    - Hypothalamus
      - Located above the pituitary gland and above the third ventricle; interacts with the pituitary gland, affecting the functions of the thyroid gland, adrenal glands, kidneys, musculoskeletal system, and reproductive organs
      - Thyrotropin-releasing hormone (TRH), gonadotropin-releasing hormone (GnRH), growth hormone-releasing hormone (GHRH), corticotropin-releasing hormone (CRH), somatostatin, and dopamine are released by the hypothalamus to the anterior pituitary (Shahid et al., 2022). Vasopressin and oxytocin are released from the hypothalamus to the posterior pituitary.
      - Syndrome of Inappropriate Anti-Diuretic Hormone (SIADH) is the result of ischemic stroke involving the hypothalamus in which there is an abnormally high level of antidiuretic hormone (ADH) released resulting in hyponatremia.

- Blood supply is from small perforating arteries off the circle of Willis
- Pituitary gland
  - Located below the hypothalamus, connected by the pituitary stalk
  - Pea-sized structure protectively encased in the bony structure, sella turcica, and composed of two distinct lobes—anterior and posterior
  - Known as the *master gland* as it controls the function of most other endocrine glands, referred to as *target glands*. Works with the hypothalamus to detect the levels of hormones produced by the target glands and releases stimulating hormones to them (Table 3.1).

Brainstem Structures: Midbrain, Pons, and Medulla Oblongata

- Midbrain, or mesencephalon
  - Uppermost portion of the brainstem; motor and sensory tracts pass through here. There are two distinct sections: the tectum and the tegmentum (see Table 3.2).
  - Blood supply is from basilar artery, PCA, and superior cerebellar artery (SCA).

TABLE 3.1

Pituitary Hormones

Anterior Lobe Hormones	Hormone Functions
ACTH, or corticotropin	Stimulates adrenal glands to produce cortisol and other hormones
FSH and LH, also referred to as gonadotropins	Stimulates ovaries to produce eggs and estrogen; testicles to produce sperm and testosterone
Growth hormone	Regulates growth and physical development; stimulates muscle formation and fat tissue reduction
Prolactin	Stimulates the mammary glands to produce milk
TSH	Stimulates the thyroid gland to produce thyroid hormones
Beta-melanocyte–stimulating hormone	Results in darkening of the skin
Enkephalins	Inhibit pain sensation
Endorphins	Reduce pain and stress; improve mood
Posterior Lobe Hormones	**Hormone Functions**
Oxytocin	Stimulates the uterus to contract, and milk release in the breast
Vasopressin	Regulates kidney excretion of water

ACTH, adrenocorticotropic hormone; FSH, follicle-stimulating hormone; LH, luteinizing hormone; TSH, thyroid-stimulating hormone.

TABLE 3.2

Midbrain Functional Areas

Midbrain Tectum	Tectum Functions
Superior colliculus	Process and transmit visual signals from the retina to the occipital lobe
Inferior colliculus	Process and transmit auditory signals from the ear through the thalamus to the temporal lobe
Midbrain Tegmentum	**Tegmentum Functions**
Reticular formation	Arousal, consciousness, sleep–wake cycles, coordination of certain movements, and cardiovascular control
PAG matter	Processes pain signals, autonomic function, and behavioral responses to fear and anxiety; may help to control defensive reactions in PTSD
Cranial nerve III—oculomotor nerve	Controls pupil and most eye movements
Cranial nerve IV—trochlear nerve	Controls eye movement down and in toward the nose
Spinothalamic tract	Transmits sensory information about pain and temperature to the thalamus
Corticospinal tract	Transmits motor information from the brain to the spinal cord
Red nucleus	Coordination of motor function
SN	Produces dopamine; relays information for control of motor function; considered part of the basal ganglia
VTA	Also produces dopamine, key to the reward system

PAG, periaqueductal gray; PTSD, posttraumatic stress disorder; SN, substantia nigra; VTA, ventral tegmental area.

  - Midbrain infarction results in impaired consciousness, eye movement disorders, hemiparesis, and ataxia.
- Pons, or metencephalon
  - Located inferior to the midbrain and superior to the medulla; motor and sensory fibers pass through here. There are two sections: dorsal pons and ventral pons (Table 3.3).
  - Blood supply is from branches of the vertebral artery and the basilar artery.
  - Pontine infarction results in double vision, vertigo, dizziness, ataxia, and in rare cases, locked-in syndrome, in which cognition is intact, but paralysis of entire body except eye movements (Rahman & Tadi, 2022).

TABLE 3.3

Pons Functional Areas

Dorsal Pons	Dorsal Pons Functions
Reticular formation	Arousal, consciousness, sleep–wake cycles, coordination of certain movements, and cardiovascular control
Ventral Pons	**Ventral Pons Functions**
Pontine nuclei	Innervated by the cerebral cortex, provide input to the cerebellum

TABLE 3.4

Medullary Functional Areas

Medullary Areas	Functions
Cardiovascular-respiratory regulation system	Regulates cardiac rhythm, blood pressure, and respiratory drive
Descending motor tracts	Carry motor information from the cerebral cortex
Ascending sensory tracts	Carry sensory information to the cerebral cortex
Origin of cranial nerves IX, X, XI, XII	IX: taste, gag, and saliva production
	X: autonomic nerve function—heart rate, intestinal activity, swallowing, and voice
	XI: muscles of neck and back
	XII: muscles of the tongue

- Medulla
  - Located below the pons; serves as connection with the spinal cord; crossover of most motor nerves occurs at level of the medulla; comprised of various functional areas (see Table 3.4)
  - Blood supply is the vertebral arteries
  - Lateral medullary infarction results in:
    - Paralysis: inability to feel temperature or pain in parts of the body, dysphagia, nausea, and vomiting
    - Wallenberg syndrome: sensory deficits affecting the trunk (torso) and extremities on the opposite side of the infarction, and sensory deficits affecting the face and cranial nerves on the same side with the infarct
    - Horner syndrome: ptosis, meiosis, and anhydrosis (Figure 3.6)

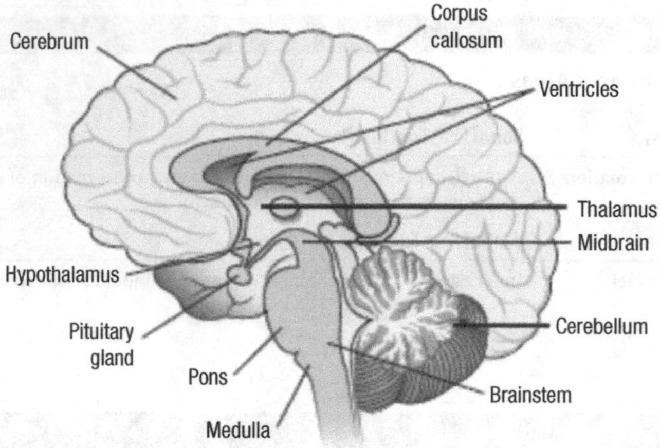

Figure 3.6 Midbrain, pons, and medulla.

Source: Morrison, K. (2023). *Stroke nursing certification review*. Springer Publishing Company.

Cerebellum

- Located in the posterior cranial fossa, behind the fourth ventricle, the pons, and the medulla oblongata, and below the posterior cerebrum (Jimsheleishvili & Dididze, 2022); separated from the cerebrum by the tentorium cerebelli, an extension of the dura mater; composed of two hemispheres with various regions of function (see Table 3.5 and Figure 3.7).
- Blood supply is the SCA, the anterior inferior cerebellar artery (AICA), and the posterior inferior cerebellar artery (PICA).
- Cerebellar infarction results in jerky, uncoordinated motor movements, known as ataxia.

Cerebellar Peduncles

- Arise from the brainstem at the level of the pons and connect through the anterior cerebellum; contain nerve fibers (efferent and afferent) that connect the cerebellum to the brainstem. There are three functional areas (see Table 3.6 and Figure 3.8).
- Blood supply is the SCA, the AICA, and the PICA.

Brain Vasculature

- The brain's entire blood supply originates from the aortic arch (see Figure 3.9).
- The circle of Willis is comprised of the internal carotid arteries (ICAs), anterior cerebral arteries (ACAs), anterior communicating artery, posterior communicating artery, and PCAs (see Figure 3.10).

TABLE 3.5

Cerebellar Functional Areas

Cerebellar Regions	Functions
Cerebrocerebellum	Receives input from the cerebral cortex, facilitates motor planning
Spinocerebellum	Receives information from the spinal cord regarding limb position and sensation; motor execution
Vermis	Facilitates upright posture, motor execution, limb and eye movement
Vestibulocerebellum	Facilitates fluidity in balance and posture, and eye movements

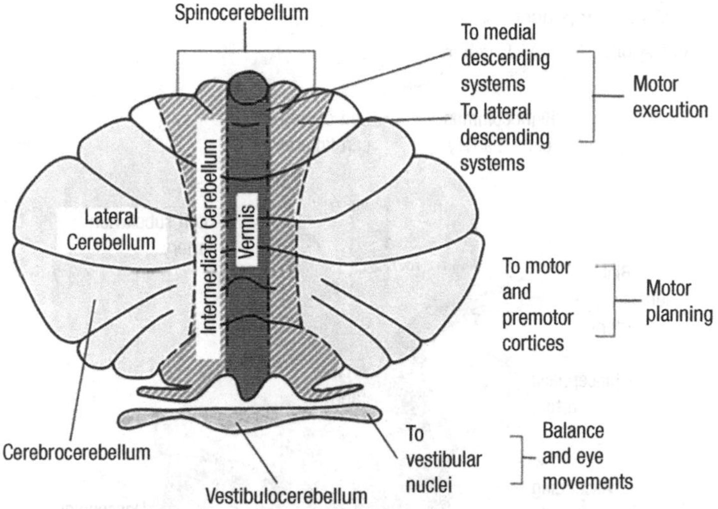

Figure 3.7 Cerebellar functional regions.

Source: Courtesy of Nicholas McLaughlin.

TABLE 3.6

Cerebellar Peduncles

Peduncle	Functions
Superior	Carries efferent signals from the cerebellum to the red nuclei and thalamus; creates feedback loop with the cerebral motor cortex
Middle	Carries afferent signals from various areas of the brain; information regarding types of voluntary movement planned
Inferior	Carries afferent signals from various areas of the brain; information on balance and proprioception

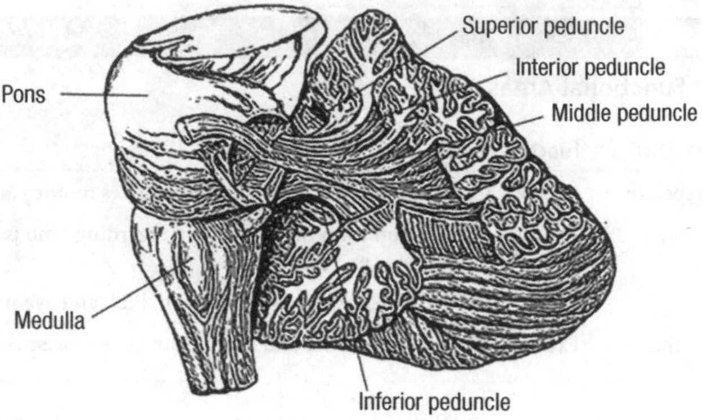

Figure 3.8 Cerebellar peduncles.

Source: Courtesy of Nicholas McLaughlin.

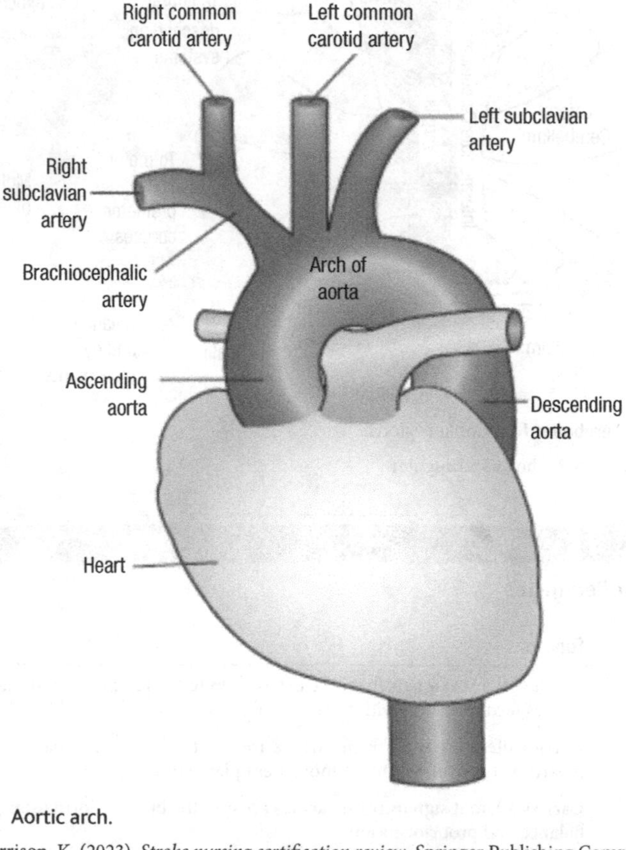

Figure 3.9 Aortic arch.

Source: Morrison, K. (2023). *Stroke nursing certification review*. Springer Publishing Company.

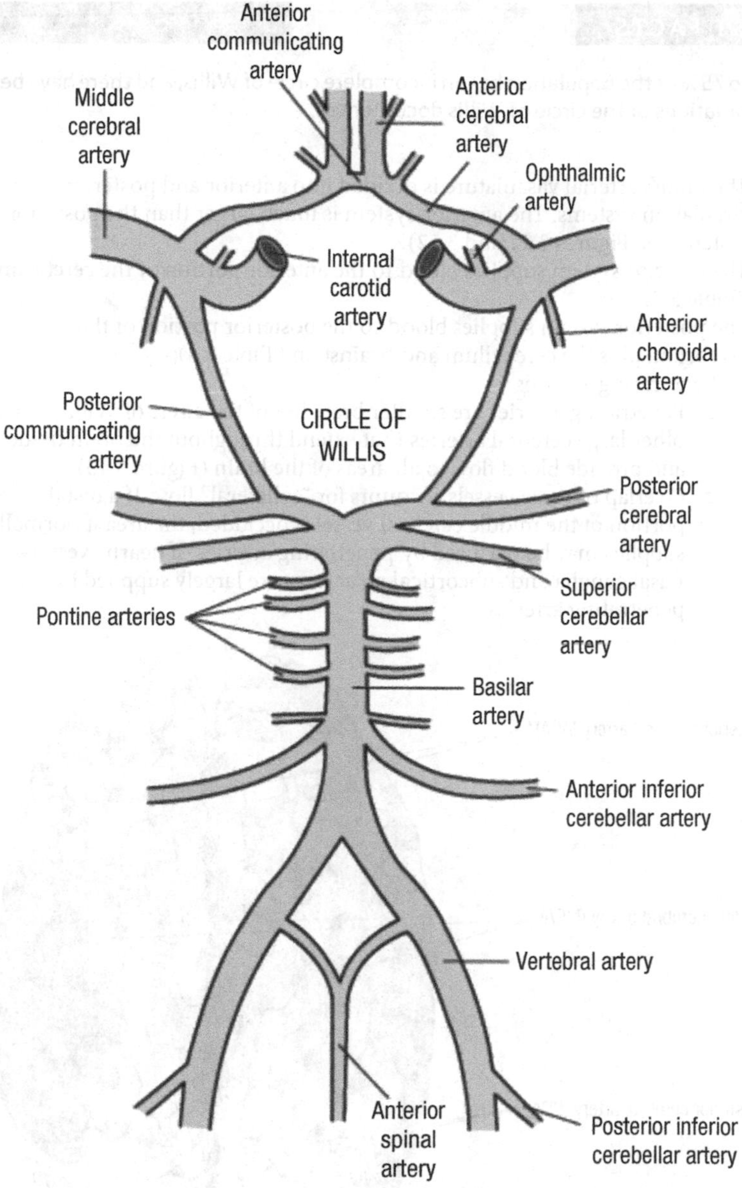

Figure 3.10 Circle of Willis.

Source: Morrison, K. (2023). *Stroke nursing certification review*. Springer Publishing Company.

FAST FACTS

Up to 75% of the population has an incomplete circle of Willis, and there have been 22 variations of the circle of Willis documented.

- The brain's arterial vasculature is divided into anterior and posterior circulation systems. The anterior system is much larger than the posterior system (see Figures 3.11 and 3.12).
- The anterior system supplies blood to the anterior portion of the cerebrum (Table 3.7).
- The posterior system supplies blood to the posterior portion of the cerebrum, plus the cerebellum and brainstem (Table 3.8).
  - Penetrating arteries
    - Penetrating arteries are smaller branches of the circle of Willis and other large cerebral arteries that extend throughout the brain tissue and provide blood flow to all areas of the brain (Figure 3.13).
    - Overlap of these vessels accounts for "collateral" flow. If a distal portion of the middle cerebral vessel is occluded, the area it normally supplies may be perfused by penetrating arteries of nearby vessels.
    - Basal ganglia and subcortical structures are largely supplied by penetrating arteries.

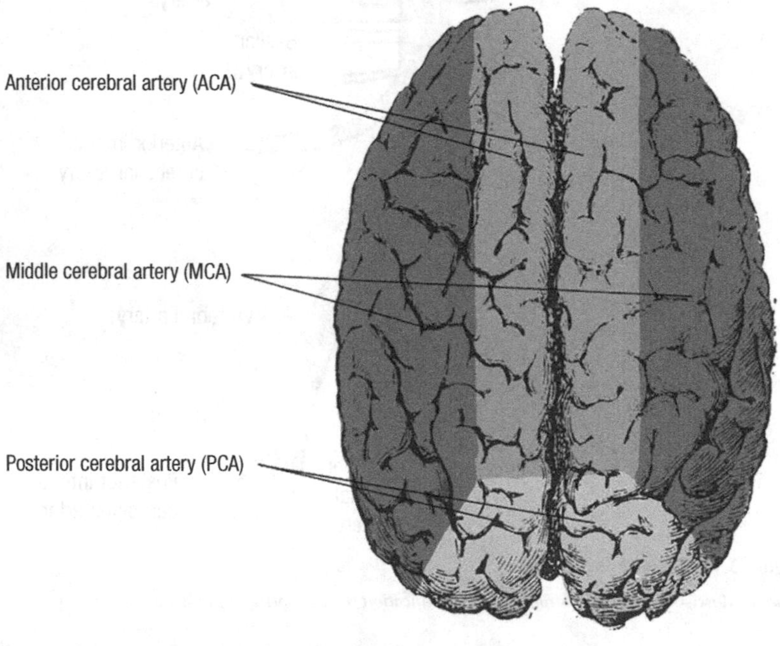

Figure 3.11 Large vessel territories superior view.

Source: Courtesy of Nicholas McLaughlin.

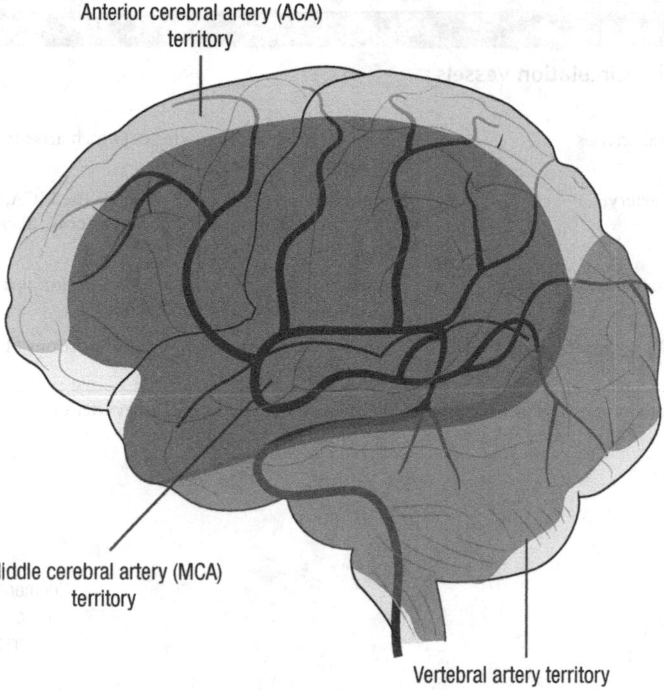

Figure 3.12 Large vessel territories lateral view.

Source: Morrison, K. (2023). *Stroke nursing certification review*. Springer Publishing Company.

TABLE 3.7

Anterior Circulation Vessels

Interial carotid arteries	Connect aorta and anterior brain vessels
Middle cebrebral arteries	Supply blood to most of frontal and parietal lobes, and lateral portion of temporal lobes, the internal capsule, and the basal ganglia
Anterior cerebral arteries	Supply blood to the medial portion of the frontal lobe, the medial and superior portions of the parietal lobes, and portions of the corpus callosum, basal ganglia, and internal capsule
Anterior communicating artery	Connects the left and right anterior cerebral arteries

TABLE 3.8

Posterior Circulation Vessels

Vertebral arteries	Connect the subclavian arteries (which arise from the aorta) and the posterior brain
Basilar artery	Supplies blood to the cerebellum via the PICA, the AICA, and the superior cerebellar arteries; also supplies blood to the pons
Posterior cerebral arteries	Supply blood to the occipital lobe, inferior portion of the temporal lobe, and the thalamus
Posterior communicating arteries	Connect the anterior and posterior portions of the circle of Willis

AICA, anterior inferior cerebellar arteries; PICA, posterior inferior cerebellar arteries.

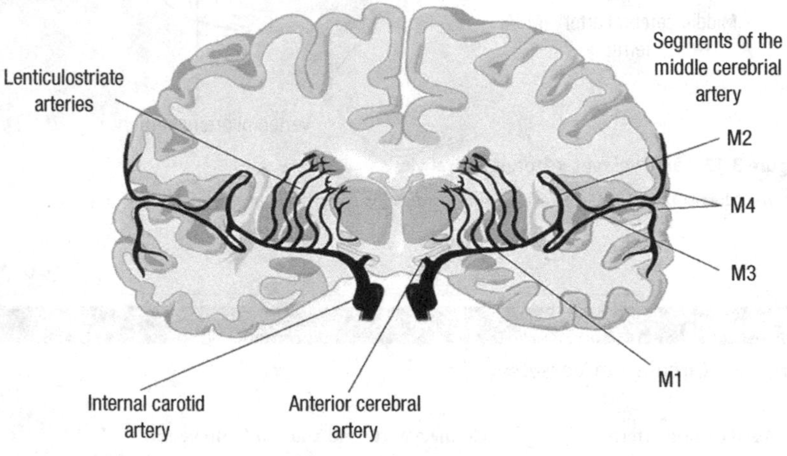

Figure 3.13 Lenticulostriate vessels and branches of MCA.

Source: Courtesy of Nicholas McLaughlin.

- Cerebral venous circulation
  - Cerebral venous circulation serves as the brain's drainage system.
  - The venous sinuses collect the blood from the brain and empty it into the internal jugular veins.
  - Dural venous sinuses (also called dural sinuses, cerebral sinuses, or cranial sinuses) are venous channels found between layers of dura mater in the brain (Figure 3.14).

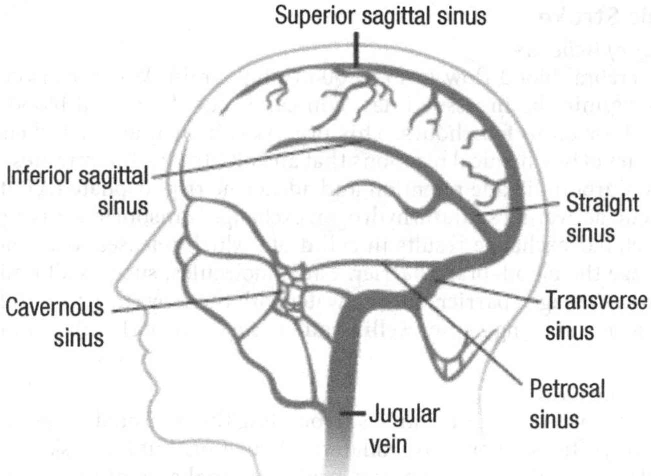

Figure 3.14 Venous system.

Source: Morrison, K. (2023). *Stroke nursing certification review*. Springer Publishing Company.

STROKE TYPES

Ischemic strokes account for 88% of all strokes due to lack of blood to part of the brain caused by narrowing or occlusion of vessels. There are two categories:

- **Thrombotic:** The vessel is narrowed or occluded due to a stationary buildup of plaque or clot.
- **Embolic:** The vessel is narrowed or occluded by a clot traveling from another vessel or the heart.

Hemorrhagic strokes account for the remaining 12% and are due to lack of blood to part of the brain caused by a ruptured blood vessel or aneurysm. There are two categories:

- **Intracerebral hemorrhage (ICH), or intraparenchymal hemorrhage (IPH):** A cerebral artery ruptures anywhere within the brain tissue.
- **Subarachnoid hemorrhage (SAH):** A cerebral artery ruptures within the subarachnoid space, most likely due to an aneurysm rupture.

FAST FACTS

Parenchyma means functional tissue—in this case brain tissue. Both intraparenchymal and ICH refer to bleeding within the brain tissue. The term IPH is becoming the preferred term over ICH as it helps eliminate the confusion with another condition that goes by the acronym ICH—intracranial hemorrhage, which refers to any bleeding within the cranium.

Ischemic Stroke

Physiology of Ischemia

Normal cerebral blood flow is 45 to 60 mL/100 g/min. When it drops below 18 mL/100 g/min, brain tissue infarction can occur if cerebral blood flow is unresolved for up to four hours. This process is known as the ischemic cascade, a series of biochemical reactions that are initiated within minutes of brain ischemia. Carbon dioxide retention and adenosine triphosphate (ATP) breakdown occur, activating sodium/hydrogen exchange transporters; disruption of normal cellular exchange results in cell death which releases toxic chemicals that damage the blood–brain barrier. Large molecules, such as albumin, pass through the damaged barrier, pulling water with them by the process of osmosis with the result being tissue swelling and edema—the ischemic penumbra.

Ischemic Penumbra

The ischemic penumbra is the area surrounding the infarcted tissue. The area is still viable, often supported by collateral circulation, but is at risk of proceeding to infarction, like the core of the stroke (original area of infarcted tissue). The tissue is swollen, resulting in diminished function, increased intracranial pressure (ICP), and somnolence. If the area proceeds to infarct, it is referred to as extending the stroke, because the core has now been enlarged. Resolution of edema generally occurs within 72 hours, as demonstrated by improvement of some deficits and by patients being more awake and alert. In hemorrhagic stroke, edema resolution takes longer than 72 hours.

Lacunar Stroke

A lacunar stroke is also referred to as small artery occlusion (SAO) and accounts for 25% of ischemic strokes (Gore et al., 2022).

- This type of stroke is caused by occlusion of smaller, penetrating arteries, blocking blood flow to small portions of the subcortical brain.
- Also referred to as pure motor or pure sensory stroke because the territory of infarct is so small as to only affect motor or sensory fibers, usually not both. The surrounding brain tissue often quickly takes over the function of the infarcted territory, thus the symptoms may only last a few hours.

Watershed Stroke

A watershed stroke occurs at the junction of distal fields of two nonanastomosing (nonconnecting) arterial systems (see Figure 3.15).

There are two types of watershed strokes:

- **Cortical watershed (CWS):** This type occurs between the territories of the ACA, middle cerebral artery (MCA), and PCA.
- **Internal watershed (IWS):** This stroke occurs in the white matter along and slightly above the lateral ventricle, between the deep and the superficial arterial systems of the MCA, or between the superficial systems of the MCA and ACA.

A watershed stroke is caused by systemic hypoperfusion or microemboli from carotid artery disease. For example, a patient awakens after surgery with new neuro deficit, but no evidence of an embolic source. Patients with vascular

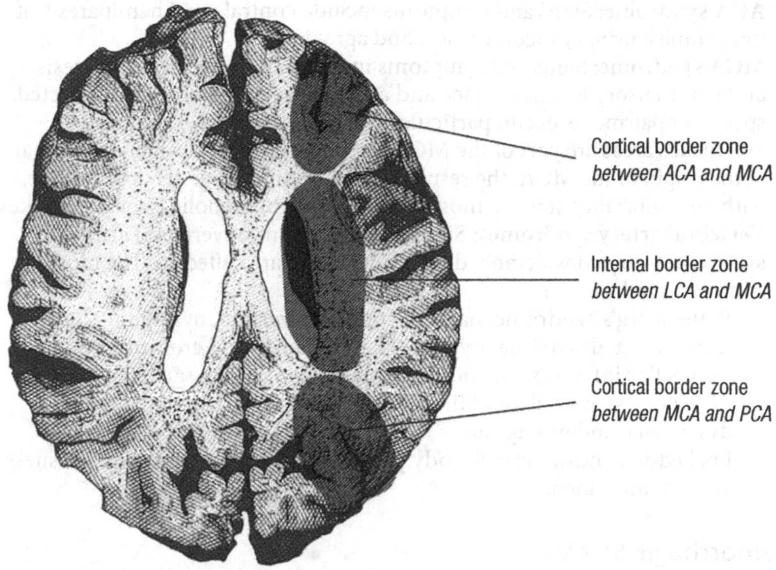

Figure 3.15 Watershed strokes.
Source: Courtesy of Nicholas McLaughlin.

disease and/or history of hypertension are less tolerant of anesthesia and resultant lower blood pressure that doesn't perfuse their distal vascular beds.

Cryptogenic Stroke

- Cryptogenic strokes account for 30% of ischemic strokes (Kamtchum-Tatuene et al., 2021).
- It is a stroke confirmed by imaging with no source found despite a thorough diagnostic workup.
- It can be further subdivided into embolic stroke of undetermined source (ESUS) or non-ESUS; in other words, if imaging confirms that the stroke is not lacunar, and no source has been found, then it is ESUS.

Large Vessel Syndromes

Large-vessel syndromes occur when the blood supply is suddenly restricted or occluded in one of the large cerebral arteries, resulting in a "syndrome" or specific set of symptoms that are often dramatic.

Large-vessel occlusions (LVO): These can be gradual, which allows collateral circulation to expand to assume the responsibility of supplying the affected region with blood, and stroke does not necessarily occur. Proximal occlusions will result in a broader set of symptoms, whereas distal occlusions will result in smaller territories of ischemia, thus a smaller set of symptoms. The incidence is thought to be up to 50% of ischemic strokes (Waqas et al., 2019).

- **ACA syndrome:** Signs and symptoms include contralateral hemiparesis of lower limbs, urinary incontinence, and apraxia.
- **MCA syndrome:** Signs and symptoms include contralateral hemiparesis and hemisensory loss in the face and arms. If the dominant side is affected, speech impairments occur, particularly aphasia, because Broca's and Wernicke's areas are part of the MCA territory. If the occlusion is proximal at the origin of the MCA, the result is a devastating, large-territory stroke, with 80% mortality. It is the most common site for embolic ischemic strokes.
- **Vertebral artery syndromes:** Signs and symptoms of vertebral artery syndromes vary considerably depending on the area affected. The most common syndromes are:
  - Wallenberg's syndrome: nausea, vomiting, vertigo, nystagmus, tachycardia, dysarthria, dysphagia, imbalance, and crossed signs
  - Cerebellar infarction: incoordination, ataxia, and dysarthria
  - PCA occlusion: unilateral limb weakness, gait ataxia, limb ataxia, dysarthria, and nystagmus
  - Locked-in syndrome: full-body paralysis with preserved consciousness and eye movement

Hemorrhagic Stroke

Hemorrhagic strokes comprise 12% of all strokes. This type of stroke occurs when a blood vessel ruptures in or near the brain, disrupting blood flow to a part of the brain. The two main types of hemorrhagic strokes are SAH and ICH (Figure 3.16).

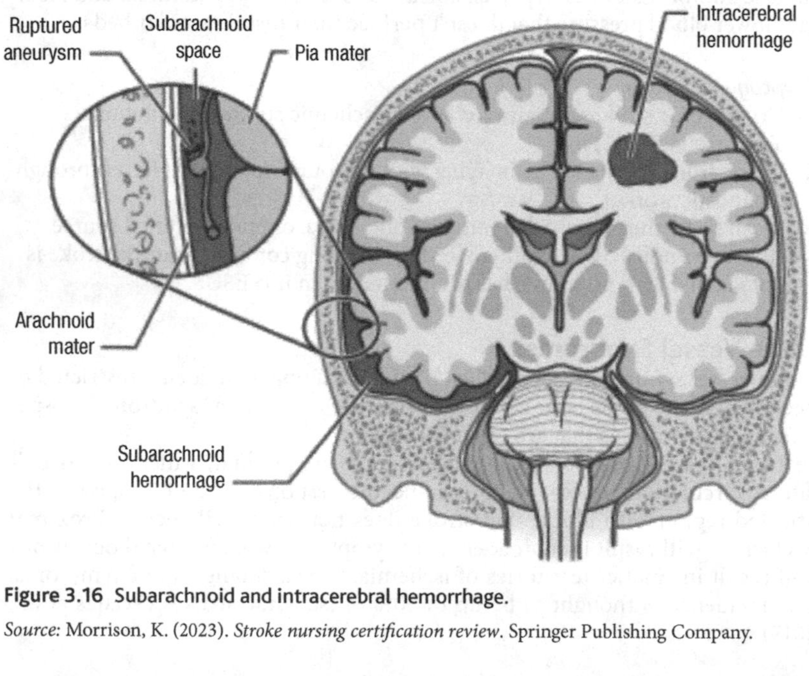

Figure 3.16 Subarachnoid and intracerebral hemorrhage.

Source: Morrison, K. (2023). *Stroke nursing certification review*. Springer Publishing Company.

TABLE 3.9

Aneurysm Types

Saccular, aka "berry," due to its shape	■ Occurs at arterial bifurcations and branches of the large arteries at the base of the brain—the circle of Willis ■ Comprises 80% to 90% of cerebral aneurysms
Fusiform	■ An outpouching of artery that is expanded in all directions, has no stem, and seldom ruptures
Dissecting	■ An aneurysm that occurs with a tear in the artery wall that separates the three layers of the wall, rather than ballooning out the entire wall

Subarachnoid Hemorrhage

- Ruptured aneurysms on large arteries are the cause of 85% of SAHs, resulting in blood collecting in the subarachnoid space. The pia mater prevents it from getting into the brain tissue (parenchyma).
- There are three types of aneurysms: saccular, fusiform, and dissecting (Florman & Ecker, 2021; Table 3.9). The most common sites for aneurysms are the anterior communicating artery, followed by the posterior communicating artery, the basilar artery, and the MCA.
- Subarachnoid blood can block circulation of cerebrospinal fluid (CSF) resulting in hydrocephalus; this usually occurs later during recovery and may appear as progressive dementia.
- Cerebral vasospasm occurs due to cerebral arteries in the subarachnoid space being surrounded by blood, which is irritating to the muscular arterial walls, resulting in spasms. Secondary ischemic stroke occurs in 30% of these patients, a condition referred to as delayed cerebral ischemia (DCI).
- Seizures occur in 7% of patients and may signal rebleeding, which occurs in 17% of patients, typically within the first 24 hours.
- Cerebral edema also develops due to SAH's effects on the blood–brain barrier, contributing to increased ICP.
- The release of catecholamines results in cardiac abnormalities, such as arrhythmias, tachycardia, and hypertension, as well as increased troponin levels.
- The mortality rate at 30 days is 40%.

Intracerebral Hemorrhage

ICH is also known as IPH.

- This type of hemorrhage is caused by rupture of a penetrating artery, which releases blood directly into the brain tissue; in essence, this is a hematoma in the brain.
- There is an inflammatory response with accompanying edema very similar to the ischemic penumbra; however, its duration is longer than that of the ischemic penumbra. The resulting increase in ICP contributes to a reduction in venous outflow, secondary ischemia (which initiates the ischemic cascade), and a breakdown of the blood–brain barrier.

- Fifty percent of ICHs occur in the basal ganglia (rupture of lenticulostriate branches of the MCA), whereas 33% occur in the cerebral hemispheres (rupture of penetrating cortical branches of the anterior, middle, and PCA).
- Hypertension is the single most important risk factor due to its dilatation of the cerebral vessels, separating the normally tight endothelial junctions of the blood–brain barrier, thus lowering the threshold for ICH. Other risk factors are anticoagulation, cigarette smoking, alcohol consumption (more than two drinks daily), cocaine or amphetamine use, malignant neoplasms, and arteriovenous malformations (AVMs).

References

Florman, J., & Ecker, R. (2021). *Neurosurgery for cerebral aneurysm*. https://emedicine.medscape.com/article/252142-overview

Gore, M., Bansal, K., Suheb, M., & Asuncion, R. (2022). *StatPearls: Lacunar stroke*. StatPearls Publishing. https://www.ncbi.nlm.nih.gov/books/NBK563216/

Jimsheleishvili, S., & Dididze, M. (2022). *StatPearls: Cerebellum neuroanatomy*. StatPearls Publishing. https://www.ncbi.nlm.nih.gov/books/NBK538167/

Kamtchum-Tatuene, J., Nomani, A., Falcione, S., Munsterman, D., Sykes, G., Joy, T., Spronk, E., Vargas, M. I., & Jickling, G. C. (2021). Non-stenotic carotid plaques in embolic stroke of unknown source. *Frontiers in Neurology*, *12*, 719329. https://doi.org/10.3389/fneur.2021.719329

Morrison, K. (2023). *Stroke nursing certification review*. Springer Publishing Company.

Rahman, R., & Tadi, P. (2022). *StatPearls: Pons neuroanatomy*. StatPearls Publishing. https://www.ncbi.nlm.nih.gov/books/NBK560589/

Shahid, Z., Asuka, E., & Singh, G. (2022). *StatPearls: Hypothalamus physiology*. StatPearls Publishing. https://www.ncbi.nlm.nih.gov/books/NBK535380/

Torrico, T., & Munakomi, S. (2022). *StatPearls: Thalamus neuroanatomy*. StatPearls Publishing. https://www.ncbi.nlm.nih.gov/books/NBK542184/

Waqas, M., Mokin, M., Primiani, C., Rai, A., Levy, E., & Siddiqui, A. (2019). Large vessel occlusion in acute ischemic stroke patients: A dual-center estimate based on a broad definition of occlusion site. *Journal of Stroke & Cerebrovascular Disease*, *29*(2), 104504. https://doi.org/10.1016/j.jstrokecerebrovasdis.2019.104504

4

Associated Stroke Disorders and Stroke Mimics

Erin Conahan

Advanced practice providers (APPs) are often consulted when patients develop acute stroke symptoms. The APP knows that not all symptoms will be attributed to acute stroke, and in some instances other causes of symptoms are identified. These are referred to as stroke mimics. It is just as important for the underlying condition to be identified and treated. Likewise, when patients are diagnosed with stroke, it is the job of the APP to determine the etiology. It is not uncommon for stroke to be caused by undiagnosed, untreated, or inappropriately treated risk factors (including noncompliance with the treatment plan). Still, there are some strokes that are caused by problems related to the blood vessels themselves (Keigher et al., 2020). It is critical for the APP to understand the pathophysiology and treatment of these conditions to implement effective primary and secondary stroke preventative measures. This section briefly reviews these disorders and discusses how these conditions can lead to stroke.

ASSOCIATED STROKE DISORDERS

Transient Ischemic Attack

- Transient ischemic attack (TIA) is a focal neurological deficit that resolves completely without intervention, *and* there is no stroke on cerebral imaging.
- TIA is often called a mini-stroke, although by definition there is no stroke on imaging.
- MRI is the preferred imaging modality for TIA, but for patients who are unable to tolerate MRI, repeat noncontrast head CT should be repeated in 12 to 24 hours to confirm no stroke on imaging.
- TIA is a warning sign; patients need to be encouraged to seek treatment. A stroke workup to identify risk factors and implementation of secondary

prevention can decrease the likelihood of the patient experiencing a future stroke.

- Scoring tools, such as the ABCD2 Score and ABCD3-I Score, are used to calculate the patient's risk of having a stroke at 7 days, 21 days (ABCD2) or 28 days (ABCD3-I), and 90 days. Higher scores indicate higher stroke risk.

FAST FACTS

In the past, TIA had a time-based definition. (If symptoms resolved within 24 hours, it was a TIA.) With improved imaging that has shown small strokes even in cases where symptoms resolved within 24 hours, TIA has developed a tissue-based definition. (If no infarct is on 24-hour imaging, it is a TIA.)

Cerebral Venous Sinus Thrombosis

- Cerebral venous sinus thrombosis (CVST) represents less than 1% of all strokes.
- Clots in the venous system prevent cerebral drainage leading to increased intracranial pressure (ICP) and vascular congestion resulting in cerebral hemorrhage or infarction.
- Intracerebral hemorrhage (ICH) and seizures are common presentations, but presentation is dependent on location, whether there is an infarct or hemorrhage, age, and acute versus chronic event.
- CVST is seen most often in younger female patients related to pregnancy or oral contraception.
- Initial treatment is symptomatic management. Anticoagulation is initiated regardless of hemorrhage. There have been trials looking at endovascular approaches, but formal recommendations have not yet been published.

Carotid Artery Dissection

- Occurs when there is a tear in the vessel wall leading to blood accumulation between layers and disruption of blood flow of the *carotid or vertebral arteries* which can lead to stroke.
- It is often seen in young patients due to sports and trauma, but spontaneous dissection can be seen in patients of all ages.
- The mechanism of injury is usually related to rotation, stretching, or vessel mobility due to degenerative changes.

Antiplatelets or anticoagulation can be used to treat dissection; there is not consistent evidence to endorse one class of antithrombotic over the other.

Moyamoya

- Gets its name from the characteristic tangle of vessels seen on imaging that develops to support collateral blood flow in narrowed or occluded cerebral arteries. It is a chronic and progressive genetic condition.

- Children are most often affected, but moyamoya can be seen in adults as well.
- Symptoms vary from person to person and can include intellectual disability (children), TIAs, or seizures.
- Treatment is symptomatic and can include medicine or surgical approaches. Primary and secondary stroke prevention are essential to maintain adequate cerebral perfusion.

Hypercoagulable State

- Workup is reserved for patients who do not have identifiable cardiovascular risk factors despite exhaustive testing.
- The most common clotting disorders are Factor V Leiden, Protein S and C deficiencies, antiphospholipid antibodies, and elevated homocysteine levels.
- CT of the chest, abdomen, and pelvis may reveal a previously undiagnosed malignancy. Cancer is known to promote clotting, and if a clot reaches the brain a stroke occurs.
- Pregnancy is a self-limiting hypercoagulable state that, in rare cases, increases stroke risk in females. Testing may reveal an underlying treatable condition. Future pregnancies may not be affected.
- Regardless of the cause, treatment is aimed at the underlying condition to prevent future stroke.

Amyloid Angiopathy

- Refers to protein deposits in small vessel walls making them weak and prone to hemorrhage.
- Similar protein deposits are seen in patients with Alzheimer disease.
- More common in older patients with cognitive impairment or dementia.
- Microhemorrhages are often seen on MRI.
- Antiplatelets and anticoagulants are usually avoided to prevent catastrophic hemorrhage.

Vasculitis

- An inflammation of blood vessels which causes vessel narrowing that can lead to stroke.
- Workup includes a thorough medical history, review of symptoms, rheumatologic and inflammatory markers, and, in some cases, tissue biopsy. Infection must be ruled out.
- There are many types of vasculitis, and treatment depends on the identified cause. Steroids or immunosuppressive agents may be used and titrated as inflammation is controlled.

Other Vascular Anomalies

- Arteriovenous malformations (AVMs) occur when there is an absence of capillaries connecting the arteries and veins. As the AVMs grow, patients can develop neurologic symptoms. Patients may present with ICH or seizures. AVMs are often congenital and may be incidental findings on cerebral imaging. Primary management is symptomatic treatment. Long-term treatment includes surgery, embolization, or radiosurgery.

- Arteriovenous fistulas (AVFs) are abnormal connections between an artery and a vein occurring in the dura. Dural AVFs are usually acquired through a thrombosed vessel, trauma, or previous craniotomy. Patients are at risk for intracranial hypertension and ischemic or hemorrhagic stroke. As with AVMs, AVFs can be treated by surgery, embolization, or radiosurgery.
- Cavernous angioma is a slow flow state marked by a series of abnormal capillaries. Cavernous angiomas are congenital conditions. Patients may develop headache, seizure, or hemorrhage. Cavernous angiomas are treated with medical management or radiosurgery.

FAST FACTS

Initiatives focused on decreasing door to needle times have resulted in an increased chance of treating stroke mimics (Pohl et al., 2021).

STROKE MIMICS

Stroke mimics refer to patients that present with symptoms of stroke that after further investigation are determined to be from nonvascular causes (Table 4.1).

- In a comprehensive research review, Pohl et al. (2021) estimated ~25% of patients presenting with stroke symptoms end up with a nonstroke diagnosis. Quantification is difficult due to various definitions used in clinical trials.
- IV alteplase treatment rates vary from 3.5% (Ali-Ahmed et al., 2019) to 17% (Pohl et al., 2021).
- Despite risk of hemorrhage with IV alteplase, rates of intracranial hemorrhage in stroke mimics are <1% (Ali-Ahmed et al., 2019; Pohl et al., 2021).

Common Symptoms Seen in Stroke Mimics

- Vertigo and dizziness
- Altered level of consciousness
- Speech disturbances
- Weakness
- Headache

Common Characteristics of Patients Presenting With Stroke Mimics

- Low National Institutes of Health Stroke Scale (NIHSS) score
- Young
- Female
- Able to ambulate
- Less likely to have classic stroke risk factors

TABLE 4.1

Clinical Characteristics Differentiating Stroke From Mimics

Characteristic	Stroke	Mimics
Age and sex	Older age (male = female)	Younger age (females > males)
Level of consciousness	Awake	Altered level of consciousness
Onset and progress	Acute and sudden	Gradual in onset
Symptom severity	Severe at onset	Fluctuations in severity are common
Risk factors	Vascular risk factors	Migraine, seizure, and systemic illness
Vascular territory	Vascular syndromes	No vascular distribution
Blood pressures at presentation	Increased blood pressure at onset is common	Blood pressure usually not increased
Signs and symptoms	Weakness (pyramidal distribution), aphasia, and visual field defects	Sensory, vertigo (dizziness), and visual
Involuntary movements	Uncommon	May have involuntary movements
Imaging	Imaging shows ischemic lesions	Imaging helpful in diagnosis
EEG	EEG may show slowing over the affected area	May show spike and wave in seizures Unilateral facial twitching and lip-smacking Giveaway weakness Arm drift/abrupt fall without pronation

Source: Buck, B. H., Akhtar, N., Alrohimi, A., Khan, K., & Shuaib, A. (2021). Stroke mimics: Incidence, aetiology, clinical features and treatment. *Annals of Medicine*, *53*(1), 420–436. https://doi.org/10.1080/07853890.2021.1890205

Final Diagnoses Once Stroke Is Ruled Out

- Seizures
- Complicated migraine
- Conversion/functional disorders
- Bell's palsy
- Electrolyte or metabolic disturbance, including recrudescence (Buck et al., 2021)
- Altered mental status (most common stroke mimic in hospitalized patients [Nouh et al., 2022])

TIPS FOR ASSESSMENT AND DIAGNOSIS

- **Vertigo/dizziness:** Thorough history including timing of vertigo (consistent, episodic, how long each episode lasts) as well as any exacerbating factors (triggers). Isolated dizziness is rarely caused by stroke.
  - "Dizzy plus" screening to assess for presence of brainstem symptoms

        - Diplopia
        - Dysarthria
        - Dysphagia
        - Dystaxia
    - Targeted physical assessment based on history
        - HINTS (head impulse-nystagmus-test of skew) exam (Pohl et al., 2021)
        - Dix-Hallpike maneuver
        - Assess for hearing loss associated with anterior inferior cerebellar artery (AICA), Meniere disease, or labyrinthitis (Pohl et al., 2021).
        - Diagnostics should be guided by information gathered from history and findings on physical assessment.
- **Seizures:** Assess for history of seizure or previous stroke; review of medications may be helpful. Interview witnesses to describe what the event looked like: abnormal movements, incontinence, tongue biting; Todd's paralysis.
- **Complicated migraine:** Assess for history of migraine; review symptoms: aura, headache; "positive" symptoms: paresthesia or visual symptoms.
- **Bell's palsy:** Assess forehead and eye movements: if a patient with drooping lower face can wrinkle their forehead and squeeze eyes shut, a pattern known as central facial weakness, it is stroke, not Bell's Palsy.
- **Electrolyte or metabolic disturbance:** Review labs: hypoglycemia, hyponatremia, and hypokalemia (Pohl et al., 2021); intoxication: alcohol or drug use.
- Conversion/functional disorders:
    - Atypical, fluctuating symptoms, inconsistent findings
    - Giveaway weakness is often related to patient effort. The extremity may initially be raised, sometimes requiring encouragement, but has a sudden collapse with minimal or no touch by the examiner.
    - Assess for Hoover's sign.
    - Assess for triggering event (Moulin & Leys, 2019).
    - History: psychiatric
    - Prognosis for recovery is not good (Pohl et al., 2021).

FAST FACTS

When evaluating a patient with stroke-like symptoms, don't forget to do the following:

- Evaluate for cortical findings on assessment.
- Review MRI diffusion weighted imaging (DWI).
- Consider access to stroke expertise: use of telestroke.
- Use scales such as recognition of stroke in the emergency room (ROSIER) or telestroke mimic score (TM-score; Buck et al., 2021).

IMPACT OF INCORRECT DIAGNOSIS ON PATIENTS

- Unnecessary treatment and expense
- Risks associated with treatment
- Diagnosis may be carried throughout record
- More likely to discharge home and able to ambulate independently at discharge (Ali-Ahmed et al., 2019)

IMPACT OF INCORRECT DIAGNOSIS ON HEALTH SYSTEMS

Buck et al. (2021) describe the implications of misdiagnosis of acute stroke, including:

- Unnecessary admissions
- Higher level of care required for monitoring
- Cost of hyperacute investigations
- Stroke center resources
- Delayed diagnosis and treatment of true problem

STROKE CHAMELEONS

Although this chapter focuses on stroke mimics, it is important to mention stroke chameleons. While stroke mimics are false positives, stroke chameleons are false negatives (Moulin & Leys, 2019). In other words, stroke chameleons are patients who present with vague or atypical symptoms that are later found to be stroke positive. These symptoms include vertigo and dizziness, headache, altered mental status, nausea/vomiting, and posterior circulation signs (Moulin & Leys, 2019). Misdiagnosis or delayed diagnosis decreases the chance of patients receiving acute stroke treatment. It also may lead to inadequate risk factor workup and inappropriate secondary prevention, contributing to worse patient outcomes (Moulin & Leys, 2019).

References

Ali-Ahmed, F., Federspiel, J. J., Liang, L., Xu, H., Sevilis, T., Hernandez, A. F., Kosinski, A. S., Prvu Bettger, J., Smith, E. E., Bhatt, D. L., Schwamm. L. H., Fonarow, G. C., Peterson, E. D., & Xian, Y. (2019). Intravenous tissue plasminogen activator in stroke mimics: Findings from get with the guidelines–stroke registry. *Circulation: Cardiovascular Quality and Outcomes*, *12*(8), e005609. https://doi.org/10.1161/circoutcomes.119.005609

Buck, B. H., Akhtar, N., Alrohimi, A., Khan, K., & Shuaib, A. (2021). Stroke mimics: Incidence, aetiology, clinical features and treatment. *Annals of Medicine*, *53*(1), 420–436. https://doi.org/10.1080/07853890.2021.1890205

Keigher, K. M., Livesay, S. K., & Wessol, J. L. (2020). *Comprehensive review for stroke nursing* (2nd ed.). American Association of Neuroscience Nurses.

Moulin, S., & Leys, D. (2019). Stroke mimics and chameleons. *Current Opinion in Neurology*, *32*(1), 54–59. https://doi.org/10.1097/WCO.0000000000000620

Nouh, A., Amin-Hanjani, S., Furie, K. L., Kernan, W. N., Olson, D. M., Testai, F. D., Alberts, M. J., Hussain, M. A., & Cumbler, E. U. (2022). Identifying best practices to improve evaluation and management of in-hospital stroke: A scientific statement from the American Heart Association. *Stroke*, *53*(4), e165–e175. https://doi.org/10.1161/STR.0000000000000402

Pohl, M., Hesszenberger, D., Kapus, K., Meszaros, J., Feher, A., Varadi, I., Pusch, G., Tibold, A., & Feher, G. (2021). Ischemic stroke mimics: A comprehensive review. *Journal of Clinical Neuroscience*, *93*, 174–182. https://doi.org/10.1016/j.jocn.2021.09.025

5

SECTION III: DIAGNOSTICS AND ASSESSMENT

Neurological and Functional Assessment in Stroke

Martina M. Kittle and Randheer Yadav

The neurological assessment is key to accurate diagnosis and prompt treatment for the stroke patient. A concise, yet thorough, neurological examination can decrease stroke intervention times resulting in improved patient outcomes. An overview of vascular territories, basic components of a neurological examination, and common stroke scales is outlined in this chapter. The information provides the advanced practice provider (APP) with foundational knowledge to quickly identify neurological conditions and improve efficiency as they assess the stroke patient.

COMPONENTS OF A NEUROLOGICAL EXAM

The following six components are fundamental to a neurological assessment. Each concept is discussed in greater detail throughout the chapter as it pertains to the evaluation of a stroke patient. Understanding these basic components can help to organize the examination and documentation of the findings.

- Mental status
  - Level of consciousness (LOC)
  - Orientation
  - Speech
- Motor
  - Strength testing
  - Muscle tone
  - Voluntary and involuntary movements
  - Tremors
  - Drift
- Sensory
  - Light touch (dull vs. sharp)
  - Pain

- Vibration
- Temperature
- Extinction
- Cortical sensation (graphesthesia and stereognosis)

- Coordination
  - Rapid alternating movements
  - Heel to shin
  - Finger to nose
  - Gait
- Cranial nerves (CN; divided into location of nerve origination)
  - Forebrain
    - CN I olfactory: ability to smell
  - Midbrain
    - CN II optic: vision
    - CN III oculomotor: eye opening, eye movements (up and down), accommodation, open eyelids, and pupillary constriction
    - CN IV trochlear: eye movements (down and inward)
  - Pons
    - CN V trigeminal: facial sensation, taste, and chewing
    - CN VI abducens: eye movements (lateral)
    - CN VII facial: facial movement/expressions, close eyelids, taste, and salivation
    - CN VIII vestibulocochlear: hearing and balance
  - Medulla
    - CN IX glossopharyngeal: sensation and taste of posterior tongue, gag reflex, salivation, and swallowing
    - CN X vagus: cough, vocal cord movement
    - CN XI spinal accessory: head rotation and shoulder shrug
    - CN XII hypoglossal: tongue movement and strength
- Reflexes

For the topic of acute stroke assessment, only pertinent reflexes are discussed here. When assessing a stroke patient who is unresponsive or comatose, knowing a few reflexes can help distinguish between a neurological event or a systemic issue such as hypoxia, infection, and so forth.

- **Posturing reflexes:** The presence of posturing is due to severe injury or compromise of the brain stem and is associated with coma. The two types of posturing are decorticate (flexor posturing) and decerebrate (extensor posturing).
- **Triple flexion:** Triple flexion is dorsiflexion of the ankle and flexion of the hip and knee. Identification of this reflex is important as it can be mistaken for withdrawal of painful stimuli. Differentiating between purposeful withdrawal and triple flexion is a valuable assessment skill in the patient with severe neurologic injury.
- **Cranial nerve reflexes:** These reflexes are commonly used in acute stroke assessment: cough (CN X), gag (CN IX and X), and corneal and facial grimacing (CN V and VII).
- **Frontal release sign:** This is the reemergence of primitive reflexes and occurs when there is an injury to the frontal lobe. In the setting of an

anterior cerebral artery (ACA) stroke, there can be reemergence of the grasp reflex (see ACA examination findings below).

BASIC NEUROVASCULAR ANATOMY AND EXAMINATION FINDINGS

Understanding the vascular territories and their functions will enable the APP to not only identify a stroke, but to also identify the anatomical location that is being infarcted (Blumenfeld, 2010).

Middle Cerebral Artery

The middle cerebral artery (MCA) is the largest vascular territory in the cerebrum and is the most common location for large vessel strokes. The MCAs are divided into three regions: superior division, inferior division, and deep territory. A large or complete territory MCA stroke is known as a *stem* or *malignant* stroke and would include the following findings based on laterality.

Left Middle Cerebral Artery Syndrome

- Right hemiparesis or hemiplegia, right hemianesthesia, right homonymous hemianopia, global aphasia, and left gaze preference.

Right Middle Cerebral Artery Syndrome

- Left hemiparesis or hemiplegia, left hemianesthesia, left homonymous hemianopia, left hemineglect, and right gaze preference. Due to profound hemineglect, patients having a right MCA stroke may be unaware of their deficits and will not recognize the left side of their body as their own.

Anterior Cerebral Artery

The ACA territory is the least common region of large vessel strokes. ACA strokes can be initially mistaken as an MCA stroke; however, there are a couple of key exam findings that set the two territories apart: (a) contralateral leg weakness as opposed to full hemiparesis including the arm and leg, and (b) abulia, an absence of motivation that can be manifested by lack of speech initiation and verbal responses. Often, the patient will be mute, making it difficult or impossible to decipher between aphasia and abulia. In addition to these, there are specific findings based on laterality as follows.

Left Anterior Cerebral Artery

- Right leg weakness, cortical sensory loss, reemergence of grasp reflex, abulia. Although not as common, left ACA strokes can have full right hemiplegia and transcortical aphasia (aphasic with repetition intact).

Right Anterior Cerebral Artery

- Left leg weakness, cortical sensory loss, reemergence of grasp reflex, abulia. Although not as common, right ACA strokes can have full left hemiplegia and left hemineglect.

Posterior Circulation and Exam Findings

Posterior Circulation Artery

- Contralateral homonymous hemianopia, visual hallucinations, memory deficits, receptive aphasia

Vertebrobasilar Artery Syndrome

- Quadriplegia, locked-in syndrome, contralateral facial palsy, ipsilateral facial numbness, nausea and vomiting (N/V), ataxia, dysarthria/dysphagia
  - It is important to rule out other causes of a poor neurological exam such as postictal phase following seizure, central nervous system infection, tumors, toxic-metabolic disturbances, and hypo/hyperglycemia.
  - Remember that a patient with locked-in syndrome will appear comatose but is awake. To evaluate for locked-in syndrome, ask the patient to blink and move their eyes vertically.

Posterior Inferior Cerebellar Artery

The posterior inferior cerebellar artery (PICA) is the most common region of cerebellar strokes and is the vessel involved in lateral medullary syndrome (also known as Wallenberg syndrome). Common symptom manifestation consists of vertigo, N/V, ipsilateral Horner syndrome, ipsilateral ataxia, nystagmus, dysphagia (often severe), dysphonia, and dysarthria. Patients may also have loss of pain and temperature sensation on the ipsilateral face and contralateral trunk and limbs. The HINTS (acronym standing for **H**ead **I**mpulse, **N**ystagmus, **T**est of **S**kew) exam can be superior to MRI in detecting central (such as PICA strokes) versus peripheral lesions. HINTS testing consists of the following:

- **Head impulse testing:** Quickly move the patient's head while patient has gazed fixed on an object (can use examiner's nose). If the patient does not have large beats of nystagmus while attempting to remain fixated on the object, there is concern for central lesion/stroke.
- **Direction-changing nystagmus:** Have patient follow finger to lateral gaze positions. Positive central finding is "bidirectional nystagmus," which is any change of nystagmus direction (vertical or horizontal) associated with lateral gaze.
- **Vertical skew:** Cover one eye, uncover quickly, positive finding of central lesion is downward position of covered eye when uncovered.

Anterior Inferior Cerebellar Artery

Anterior inferior cerebellar artery (AICA) strokes are also called lateral pontine syndrome and have similar presentation as PICA with a few exceptions such as ipsilateral hearing loss, facial paralysis, loss of pain/temperature sensation, loss of taste from anterior portion of the tongue, and decreased lacrimation and salivation. Other manifestations are consistent with PICA strokes including N/V, vertigo, ataxia, and ipsilateral Horner syndrome.

Wrong-Way Eyes

Pontine strokes can have gaze deviation contralateral to the location of the stroke. This is often called "wrong-way eyes" as supratentorial strokes

(ACA/MCA) will have gaze deviation towards the side of the stroke (Johkura et al., 2011). For example, left MCA stroke will have left gaze deviation whereas a left pontine stroke will have a right gaze deviation. The exception to this is in the case of thalamic hemorrhages. Severe thalamic hemorrhage can present with wrong-way eyes, looking away from the side of hemorrhage or downward towards the nose (Ahmad & Kumar, 2014). The cause for this may be due to downward compression on the brainstem. Patients with this phenomenon typically have large hemorrhages and poor outcomes.

Cortical Versus Subcortical Findings

Cortical and subcortical deficits can be differentiated based on exam findings. Distinguishing between cortical and subcortical deficits helps to identify small vessel strokes versus large vessel strokes and can aid in early identification of a large vessel occlusion (LVO).

Cortical

- Aphasia
- Extinction and inattention
- Homonymous visual field defects
- Cortical sensory loss: loss of stereognosis, graphesthesia, and proprioception

Subcortical (Lacunar) Signs

- **Pure motor hemiparesis:** unilateral face, arm, and leg weakness, without sensory deficits
- **Ataxic hemiparesis:** unilateral arm and leg ataxia
- **Pure sensory:** loss of all sensation to the contralateral face and body
- **Sensorimotor stroke:** weakness and numbness of unilateral face, arm, and leg with an absence of cortical signs
- **Dysarthria-clumsy hand syndrome:** rare lacunar stroke syndrome characterized by dysarthria, dysphagia, and a weak, clumsy hand

STROKE ASSESSMENT SCALES AND SCORING

From the hyperacute to the subacute stroke phase, the assessment can detect even subtle changes and alert the provider to potential complications such as bleeding or worsening edema. There have been numerous scales and scoring systems developed to help streamline and standardize the assessment process. The most common scales will be discussed in this section as well as the advantages and disadvantages to each.

National Institutes of Health Stroke Scale

The National Institutes of Health Stroke Scale (NIHSS) is the most widely used assessment scale for acute and follow-up evaluation (Table 5.1). The NIHSS is the standard assessment tool to determine candidacy for intervention and to predict long-term outcomes. For the hospitalized patient, the NIHSS serves as an objective neurological assessment and reliable tool for close patient monitoring. For the novice stroke APP, memorizing and developing a script for the

TABLE 5.1

NIHSS Items for Stroke Evaluation

1a	LOC	(0–3 points)
1b	LOC Questions	(0–2 points)
1c	LOC Commands	(0–2 points)
2	Best Gaze	(0–2 points)
3	Visual	(0–3 points)
4	Facial Palsy	(0–3 points)
5a & 5b	Motor Arm	(0–4 points for each arm)
6a & 6b	Motor Leg	(0–4 points for each arm)
7	Limb Ataxia	(0–2 points)
8	Sensory	(0–2 points)
9	Best Language	(0–3 points)
10	Dysarthria	(0–2 points)
11	Extinction and Inattention	(0–2 points)

LOC, level of consciousness.

Source: Adapted from National Institute of Neurological Disorders and Stroke. (2013). *NIH Stroke Scale*. https://stroke.nih.gov/documents/NIH_Stroke_Scale.pdf

NIHSS can enable a rapid and accurate evaluation of the acute stroke patient. In the ED, it quantifies the severity of the deficits and facilitates communication by creating a common language among healthcare professionals. The NIHSS consists of 15 items and is the gold standard for initial stroke evaluation.

FAST FACTS

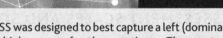

Keep in mind, the NIHSS was designed to best capture a left (dominant) hemisphere MCA stroke, giving a higher score for these patients. The greatest limitation of the NIHSS is the lack of scoring items for a posterior stroke, so while a patient may be having significant deficits from a cerebellar stroke, the NIHSS may be disproportionately low.

CHA_2DS_2-VASc Score

This score is a risk stratification score to determine the 1-year risk of stroke in a non-anticoagulated patient with nonvalvular atrial fibrillation. It is more inclusive of common stroke risk factors and modifiers than the previous version, $CHADS_2$. The acronym stands for:

- Cardiac failure
- Hypertension history
- Age >75—gets 2 points, therefore the subscript 2
- Diabetes history

- Stroke/transient ischemic attack (TIA)/thromboembolism history—gets 2 points, therefore the subscript 2
- Vascular disease history (prior myocardial infarction [MI], peripheral artery disease, or aortic plaque)
- Age 65 to 74
- Sex category—female

Score 0: All patients with atrial fibrillation will be prescribed at least an antithrombotic, while a score of 1 or greater equals a strong consideration for oral anticoagulation. If the score of 1 is due to gender alone, anticoagulant therapy is not warranted.

Glasgow Coma Scale

The Glasgow Coma Scale (GCS) is an acute evaluation, mostly used for hemorrhagic strokes. Nonspecific, the scale was originally created for evaluation of trauma patients.

Modified Rankin Score

Utilized for both acute and follow-up evaluation, the Modified Rankin Score (mRS) is used to determine functional capacity. The score ranges from 0 (no disability) to 6 (death). In the acute phase of stroke evaluation, mRS is used to determine candidacy for thrombectomy. Most institutions consider patients with an mRS of 3 or less (able to walk independently) to be a candidate for thrombectomy. This mRS range was the criteria in the **D**iffusion-Weighted Imaging or CTP **A**ssessment With Clinical Mismatch in the Triage of **W**ake-Up and Late Presenting Strokes Undergoing **N**eurointervention With Trevo (DAWN) trial, the large, randomized trial that found thrombectomy to be superior to standard care alone. However, some institutions adhere to more strict criteria of mRS of 0 or 1 for thrombectomy candidacy. The mRS is also useful in assessing long-term stroke outcomes.

ABCD2

This is a scoring tool used for TIA risk stratification. It identifies those at greatest risk of stroke for the 90 days following a TIA event. There are five components of the score: age >60, elevated blood pressure (BP), unilateral weakness or speech impairment during event, and TIA duration greater or less than 60 minutes. Scores range from 0 to 7, with the highest scores associated with higher 90-day stroke risk.

Intracerebral Hemorrhage Score

The intracerebral hemorrhage (ICH) score is used at time of presentation to provide expected mortality. The ICH score consists of GCS, ICH volume, presence of intraventricular hemorrhage (IVH), infratentorial location, and age (>80 years). The score can range from 0 (0% mortality) to 6 (100% mortality).

Max-ICH Score

Recently proven to be superior in predicting functional outcome after ICH when compared to the ICH score (Sembill et al., 2021), the Max-ICH score differs from the ICH score with inclusion of age >75, NIHSS, and use of anticoagulation. Scores range from 0 to 9.

World Federation of Neurological Surgeons

The grading scale for subarachnoid hemorrhage is a severity scale based on GCS and presence of focal motor deficit.

- **Grade 1:** GCS 15
- **Grade 2:** GCS 13 to 14, without focal deficit
- **Grade 3:** GCS 13 to 14, focal neurological deficit present
- **Grade 4:** GCS 7 to 12
- **Grade 5:** GCS 3 to 6

Modified Fisher Scale

This scale is used in aneurysmal subarachnoid hemorrhage to determine risk of symptomatic vasospasm (Table 5.2).

Hunt and Hess Scale

Used in aneurysmal subarachnoid hemorrhage and associated with risk of mortality (Table 5.3).

PREHOSPITAL SCALES

Reducing time to acute stroke intervention is a priority and should begin on initial evaluation by emergency medical services (EMS) personnel. Prehospital

TABLE 5.2

Modified Fisher Scale

Grade 1	Thin SAH (<1 mm); no IVH	24% risk of vasospasm
Grade 2	Thin SAH (<1 mm); IVH present	33% risk of vasospasm
Grade 3	Thick SAH (<1 mm); no IVH	33% risk of vasospasm
Grade 4	Thick SAH (<1 mm); IVH present	40% risk of vasospasm

SAH, subarachnoid hemorrhage; IVH, intraventricular hemorrhage.

TABLE 5.3

Hunt and Hess Scale

Grade	Characteristics		Mortality
Grade 1	Asymptomatic and mild headache	Minimal/slight nuchal rigidity	1% to 3%
Grade 2	Moderate to severe headache	Nuchal rigidity, no neurologic deficit	3% to5%
Grade 3	Drowsiness or confusion	Mild focal neurologic deficit	9% to 19%
Grade 4	Stupor	Moderate to severe hemiparesis	23% to 42%
Grade 5	Deep coma	Decerebrate rigidity	70% to 77%

scales have been added to stroke protocols to ensure hospital personnel and equipment are available upon patient arrival so that there are no delays in treatment (Pérez de la Ossa et al., 2014). There are numerous prehospital scales, and the most used are listed here.

Cincinnati Prehospital Stroke Scale

This includes scores for facial drooping, arm weakness, and speech deficits only favoring anterior stroke syndromes.

Los Angeles Prehospital Stroke Scale

This includes both physical findings of stroke (facial symmetry, grip, and arm strength) as well as screening criteria (age, baseline function, seizure history, glucose, and time of symptom onset).

Rapid Arterial Occlusion Evaluation Scale

This is a tool to identify a high probability of an LVO. Scoring criterion include facial palsy, arm and leg motor function, and aphasia. A score of 5 or greater predicts an LVO with a sensitivity of 85% and specificity of 69%.

FUNCTIONAL NEUROLOGICAL ASSESSMENT

Functional neurological disorder (FND), also known as conversion disorder, is a common stroke mimic. Patients may present with focal neurological deficits that are not fully consistent with stroke or attributable to a particular vascular territory. A suspicion of FND should not preclude a patient from receiving acute stroke intervention. Given the safety of thrombolytics and urgency of administration in the acute phase of stroke, it is best to err on the side of overtreatment if there is a possibility of stroke. There are exam techniques that can assist the APP in recognition of possible FND to guide treatment and follow-up care.

FAST FACTS

The key to a functional neurological exam is to look for inconsistency, reversibility, and symptomatology that is not consistent with a vascular territory or dermatome (Popkirov et al., 2020).

The following are quick and simple exam techniques to be familiar with.

Motor Exam

- **Hoover's sign:** This is a maneuver to evaluate for inconsistency and decreased effort with hip flexion. The examiner will ask the patient to lift the affected (weak) leg while placing a hand on the heel of the unaffected foot. A normal finding would be strong downward pressure under the unaffected foot. The absence of downward pressure shows a lack of effort and is a positive finding in FND. The examiner can perform the maneuver on both legs to notice the difference between each leg.

- **Drift without pronation:** The examiner asks for arms to be held up with supination of hands. A drift of the arm while maintaining supination of the hand would be a positive finding of FND. Drift *with* pronation is associated with upper motor neuron dysfunction and is expected in a patient with stroke.
- **Give-way weakness:** Also referred to as collapsing weakness, this is when there is inconsistent and sudden loss of tone during strength testing. Give-way weakness can be described as bouncing of the arm or leg while elevated, showing inconsistent effort. There can be false positive give-way weakness in situations where there is pain in the limb or if the patient is lethargic and being reminded of the task.
- **Hand drop test:** The hand drop test can show reversibility in a patient's weakness. The examiner will lift the patient's arm over the head/face and watch to see if the arm is lowered slowly or with intention to avoid striking the face. The examiner should be cautious with this technique, being prepared to catch the arm, as the hand could fall abruptly on the patient's face.

Sensory Exam

- Midline splitting can be tested by asking the patient to determine where the area of numbness ends/begins on the forehead. Given the overlap of cutaneous nerves, the patient will not have consistent and exact "splitting" of sensation at the center of the forehead. A finding consistent with FND would be the loss of sensation (touch or vibratory) at the center of the forehead. This finding should be considered as part of a larger functional exam as there have been organic causes of midline splitting, although this is rare.

Speech and Language

- Stuttering speech is quite common in patients who present with FND versus stroke. Again, the examiner should watch for inconsistency and reversibility. Does the patient have periods of clear speech absent of dysarthria or aphasia? The presence of grimacing and neck extension with stuttering speech is also consistent with FND clinical findings (Stone, 2005).
- Slowed and/or accented speech is also common. Understanding aphasia will help the examiner decipher between FND speech findings and stroke-related speech deficits. An aphasic patient will have difficulty producing and/or understanding language and will most commonly present with other stroke symptoms. Strokes solely causing aphasia are rare, so speech should be thoroughly assessed for signs of FND in these presentations.
- Speech symptoms that favor FND are as follows:
  - Periods of clear speech preceded by slow speech
  - The appearance that speech can only be produced with significant effort
  - Baby talk

- Broken speech
- Inability to talk but able to mouth words or write/text

A concise neurological assessment is imperative to an accurate and timely diagnosis for the patient with acute stroke. Always remember that time is brain!

Final key take-aways for acute stroke assessment include the following:

- Know the vascular territories and expected deficits for a stroke in each area. Begin learning the most common territories first—the MCA, posterior circulation artery (PCA), PICA, and subcortical territories. Then expand your knowledge from there. This knowledge will help you quickly recognize a large territory stroke and improve your confidence as an APP!
- Become familiar with the NIHSS. Have a script written or memorized to ensure efficiency and completeness. Begin with level of consciousness (LOC) and orientation questions, then move from the head (vision, gaze, and facial symmetry/sensation) and continue down the body through the extremities (ataxia, sensation, and extinction). Remember that when evaluating for possible acute stroke interventions, a comprehensive neurological exam is not indicated and will delay treatment time.
- A suspicion of FND does not make a patient ineligible for acute stroke treatments! Gather all the data and do not withhold treatment if the patient has debilitating symptoms that may be consistent with stroke.

References

Ahmad, K. E., & Kumar, K. R. (2014). "Peering at the tip of the nose" as a sign of thalamic haemorrhage. *Neuro-Ophthalmology*, *38*(1), 21–23. https://doi.org/10.3109/01658107.2013.809464

Blumenfeld, H. (2010). *Neuroanatomy through clinical cases* (2nd ed.). Sinauer Associates, Inc. Publishers.

Johkura, K., Nakae, Y., Yamamoto, R., Mitomi, M., & Kudo, Y. (2011). Wrong-way deviation: Contralateral conjugate eye deviation in acute supratentorial stroke. *Journal of the Neurological Sciences*, *308*(1–2), 165–167. https://doi.org/10.1016/j.jns.2011.06.010

Pérez de la Ossa, N., Carrera, D., Gorchs, M., Querol, M., Millán, M., Gomis, M., Dorado, L., López-Cancio, E., Hernández-Pérez, M., Chicharro, V., Escalada, X., Jiménez, X., & Dávalos, A. (2014). Design and validation of a prehospital stroke scale to predict large arterial occlusion. *Stroke*, *45*(1), 87–91. https://doi.org/10.1161/STROKEAHA.113.003071

Popkirov, S., Stone, J., & Buchan, A. M. (2020). Functional neurological disorder. *Stroke*, *51*(5), 1629–1635. https://doi.org/10.1161/STROKEAHA.120.029076

Sembill, J. A., Castello, J. P., Sprügel, M. I., Gerner, S. T., Hoelter, P., Lücking, H., Doerfler, A., Schwab, S., Huttner, H. B., Biffi, A., & Kuramatsu, J. B. (2021). Multicenter validation of the max-ICH score in intracerebral hemorrhage. *Annals of Neurology*, *89*(3), 474–484. https://doi.org/10.1002/ana.25969

Stone, J. (2005). Functional symptoms and signs in neurology: Assessment and diagnosis. *Journal of Neurology, Neurosurgery & Psychiatry*, *76*(Suppl 1), i2–i12. https://doi.org/10.1136/jnnp.2004.061655

6

Diagnostic Stroke Workup

Justin Lowe

Advanced practice providers (APPs) are often responsible for ordering the diagnostic tests for acute stroke patients. Knowledge of the recommended laboratory and imaging studies will expedite the treatment process and will ensure that the right information is available as soon as possible. Of the ever-increasing number of studies available, it is important to understand the indications for each one—not only to ensure the right information is available, but also to be cognizant of the high cost of healthcare.

LABORATORY STUDIES

- Basic laboratory workup
  - Hemoglobin A1c
  - Lipid profile
  - Complete blood count with platelets
  - Basic metabolic panel
- Additional laboratory workup based on individualized patient
  - Hypercoagulable workup
    - Arterial hypercoagulability: lupus anticoagulant, beta-2 glycoprotein, anticardiolipin antibodies, and homocysteine level
    - Venous hypercoagulability: protein C, protein S, factor V Leiden, prothrombin gene mutation, and antithrombin III

FAST FACTS

Caution to ordering labs in the acute setting of thrombosis and/or patients already on anticoagulation. Homocysteine level, beta-2 glycoprotein, and anticardiolipin antibodies are not affected, but all other studies (see section on Imaging Studies) can be unreliable in this setting.

- Lumbar puncture to evaluate cerebrospinal fluid (CSF) or infectious or inflammatory causes of stroke in certain cases
- Blood cultures if concern for bacteremia/infectious endocarditis
- Autoimmune labs such as antinuclear antibodies (ANA), erythrocyte sedimentation rate (ESR), C-reactive protein (CRP), and rheumatoid factor to evaluate for systemic inflammatory conditions that can be associated with stroke

IMAGING STUDIES

Standard Studies for Nearly All Stroke Patients

Noncontrast CT Imaging of the Brain and Vascular Imaging With Either Magnetic Resonance Angiogram or CT Angiogram

- Evaluate large vessels for occlusions, stenosis, atherosclerosis
- Also, important to obtain CT angiogram (CTA) in patients presenting with hemorrhage to assess for aneurysms, vascular malformations, and spot sign
  - Spot sign indicates continued extravasation of contrast suggesting continued hemorrhage and risk of hematoma expansion.
- CT perfusion imaging/magnetic resonance (MR) perfusion if indicated: primarily in the acute setting to determine eligibility for mechanical thrombectomy in extended time windows
- Transthoracic echocardiogram (TTE) +/− bubble study for patent foramen ovale (PFO): monitors for cardiac sources of emboli such as left atrium/atrial appendage thrombus, valvular disease, and left ventricular thrombus
- Cardiac monitoring with at least 48-hour Holter monitor: monitoring study for cardiac arrhythmias such as atrial fibrillation

Additional Supplementary Imaging/Monitoring

- **Carotid Doppler:** confirmatory testing to evaluate proximal internal carotid arteries for disease
- **Transesophageal echocardiogram (TEE):** more sensitive for detection of PFO, valvular disease, and left atrial appendage for thrombus; may also better visualize the proximal aorta and aortic arch
- Transcranial Doppler (TCD)
  - Embolic detection study: useful for carotid disease to monitor for active embolization from proximal carotid artery disease
  - Bubble study for PFO: noninvasive technique; improved sensitivity when compared to TTE
  - Stenosis study: noninvasive technique to evaluate intracranial vessels; also used for monitoring for vasospasm in subarachnoid hemorrhage
- **Lower extremity venous duplex and MR venogram pelvis studies:** used to evaluate for paradoxical emboli if PFO is present
- **MR vessel wall imaging:** may aid in distinguishing disease processes leading to intracranial arterial stenoses (vasculitis, reversible cerebral vasoconstriction syndrome, and intracranial atherosclerotic disease)

- **MR plaque morphology studies:** useful for detecting high-risk plaque features which may prompt more urgent surgical evaluation
- **Implantable loop recorder:** used for long-term evaluation for atrial fibrillation
- **Digital subtraction angiography (DSA) or catheter angiography:** detailed evaluation of vessels; can be diagnostic and treatment option; used for evaluating and treating aneurysms/vasospasm/intracranial or extracranial stenosis; more accurate in assessing for cerebral vasculitis than computed tomography angiography (CTA) or magnetic resonance angiography (MRA)

IMAGING STUDIES IN DETAIL

CT Head Without Contrast

- Measures density of tissue utilizing Hounsfield units
  - Increasing density of tissues results in increasing brightness (see Figure 6.1)
- Hemorrhage can be readily visualized
- Utilized for patient selection for acute management of ischemic stroke including intra-arterial thrombectomy as well as thrombolytic therapy
- Early signs of ischemia seen on CT
  - Hyperdense vessel sign which is suggestive of acute thrombus in a vessel
  - Early indicators if stroke/cerebral edema:
    - Loss of the insular ribbon
    - Effacement of sulci
    - Loss of gray/white matter differentiation in basal ganglia and cortical/subcortical regions

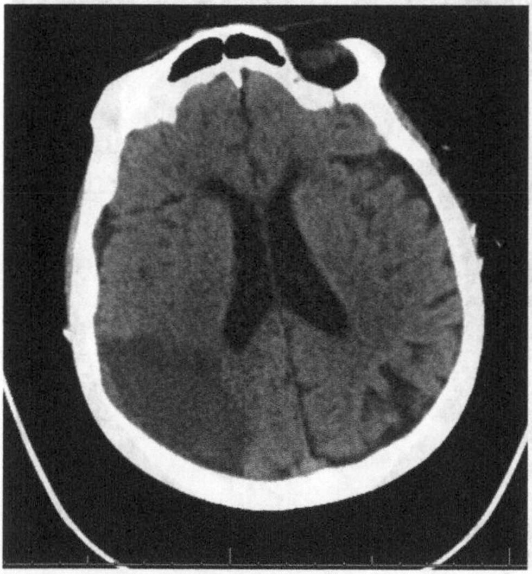

Figure 6.1 CT no contrast; ischemic stroke; axial view.
Source: Courtesy of Penn State Health Radiology Department.

- CT head and hemorrhage
  - As blood ages on CT scan the appearance will also change.
  - Blood tends to age from the outside of the hemorrhage towards the center, oftentimes creating a mixed appearance of hemorrhage.
    - Acute blood is hyperdense, subacute blood is isodense, and chronic hemorrhage is hypodense (Ermak, 2019).
    - Identifies blood in subarachnoid and intraparenchymal regions (Figures 6.2 and 6.3).
    - Blood can represent hemorrhagic conversion of ischemic stroke. Using standard terminology (HI 1, HI 2, PH 1, and PH 2) aids in defining the severity of the conversion, with PH 1 and PH 2 involving more volume of the stroke territory and being more likely to impact outcomes and be symptomatic (see Table 6.1).
- Alberta Stroke Program Early CT score (ASPECTS)
  - ASPECTS
  - Scoring system that subtracts a point for ischemic changes at 10 different areas
  - Caudate, internal capsule, and lentiform nucleus
  - At the level of the basal ganglia, three cortical regions (M1–M3) and the insular cortex
  - At the level of the ventricles just superior to the basal ganglia, three cortical regions (M4–M6; Barber et al., 2000)
  - Primarily for anterior circulation/MCA events
  - Originally used in IV tissue plasminogen activator (tPA) cases for outcome predictions (Barber et al., 2000)
  - Later included in guidelines for endovascular therapy (Powers et al., 2018)

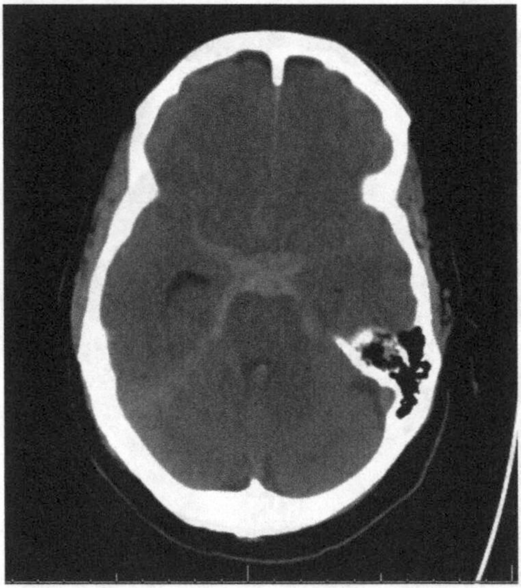

Figure 6.2 Subarachnoid hemorrhage; axial view.
Source: Courtesy of Penn State Health Radiology Department.

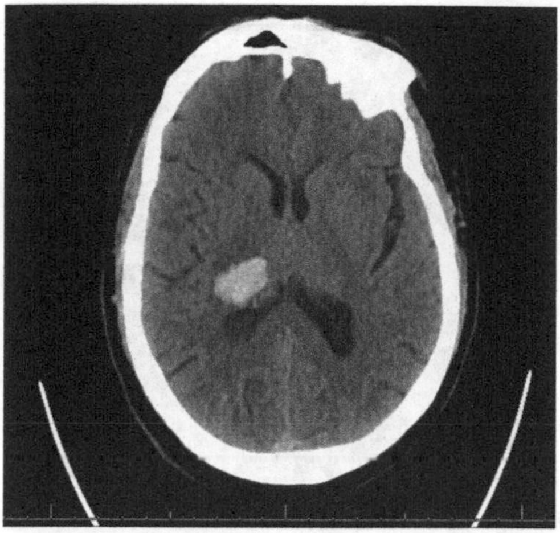

Figure 6.3 Intraparenchymal hemorrhage; axial view.
Source: Courtesy of Penn State Health Radiology Department.

TABLE 6.1

Hemorrhagic Conversion Types

HI 1	Small hyperdense petechiae
HI 2	Merging hyperdense petechiae
PH 1	Homogeneous hyperdensity occupying <30% with some mass effect
PH 2	Homogeneous hyperdensity occupying >30% with significant mass effect

HI, hemorrhagic infarction; PH, parenchymal hemorrhage.

CT Angiogram

- Uses intravenous injections of contrast dye to visualize vessels
- Provides high-quality visualization of vessels and vessel walls to include calcium deposition
- Accurate detection of degree of stenosis and can detect critical stenosis or even trickle flow
- Widely available and accessible for evaluation of vessels; first choice in hyperacute setting to evaluate for large vessel occlusion (LVO; see Figure 6.4)
- Can be used for intracranial and extracranial vessels
- Use can be limited by the following:
  - Renal disease—however, a review in 2017 revealed no increase in acute kidney injury in stroke patients that received contrast (Brinjikji et al., 2017)
  - Contrast dye allergy
  - Poor IV access since it is necessary to complete study
  - Calcium can lead to artifact or image obscuration

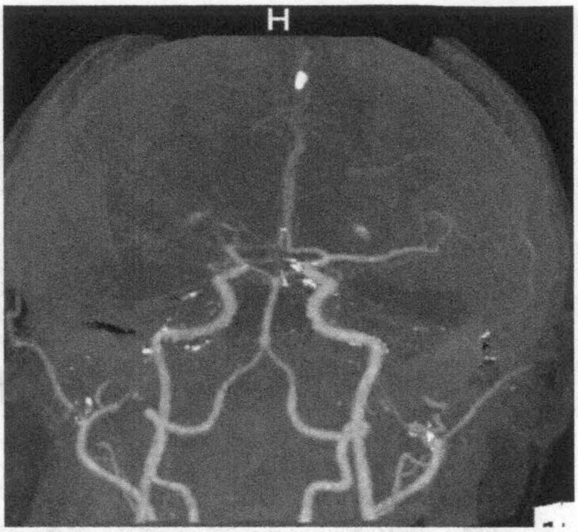

Figure 6.4 CT angio; large vessel occlusion; coronal view.

Source: Courtesy of Penn State Health Radiology Department.

CT Perfusion

- Uses a bolus injection of contrast and repeated imaging to obtain measurements of blood flow and blood flow dynamics
- Possible predictor of salvageable tissue and tissue that may be irreversibly damaged (core infarct), although several limitations:
  - Positioning/movement artifact
  - Less reliable for small strokes or posterior fossa strokes
  - Can overestimate/underestimate irreversible injury (Vagal et al., 2019)
- Four primary perfusion maps produced
  - Cerebral blood flow (CBF): measured as a rate; the volume of blood flowing through a particular volume of brain tissue per a unit of time
  - Cerebral blood volume (CBV): total volume of blood in a particular volume of brain tissue
  - Time to peak (TTP): time from when contrast injection is started to maximum contrast concentration
  - Mean transit time (MTT): average time taken for contrast to flow through a particular area of the brain (Wing & Markus, 2018)
- Uses computer processing and a mathematical algorithm to generate images (Demeestere et al., 2020)
- Useful in distinguishing stroke mimics such as migraine and seizure
- Many trials have used CT perfusion as a marker to extend the treatment windows for both endovascular therapy and thrombolytic therapy (Demeestere et al., 2020):
  - DEFUSE trial: utilized perfusion imaging to select patients for thrombectomy at six to 16 hours from last known well (Albers et al., 2018)
  - EXTEND trial: use of thrombolysis at four and a half to 9 hours based on candidacy determined by CT perfusion studies (Ma et al., 2019)
- Current guidelines recommend against using perfusion in patients within the thrombolysis window or within 6 hours from last known well time (Powers et al., 2018).

MRI

- MRI utilizes a magnet to polarize molecules, most notably of which is water.
- Radiofrequencies are emitted as molecules return to baseline.
  - Time for recovery is noted at two time points: T1 and T2 (T = time).
  - Images are obtained during the time for recovery for each time point.
  - Measured as signal intensities (hyperintense, hypointense, and isointense)
- MRI images are all based on either T1 or T2 (also known as T1 or T2 weighted; Table 6.2).
- T1 images are anatomical: gray matter appears mostly gray; white matter appears mostly white (Figure 6.5).
  - CSF is dark on T1.
  - Not used often in stroke; however, T1 images can be used in aging hemorrhage.
- T2 imaging is opposite of T1. Gray matter appears brighter and white matter is darker/gray; CSF is bright on standard T2 (Ermak, 2019; Figure 6.6).

TABLE 6.2

T1/T2/Comparison

Phase	T1	T2
Hyperacute: <12 hours	Isointense	Hyperintense
Acute: 12 hours to 2 days	Isointense	Hypointense
Early subacute: 2 to 7 days	Hyperintense	Hypointense
Late subacute: 8 to 28 days	Hyperintense	Hyperintense
Chronic: >28 days	Hypointense	Hypointense

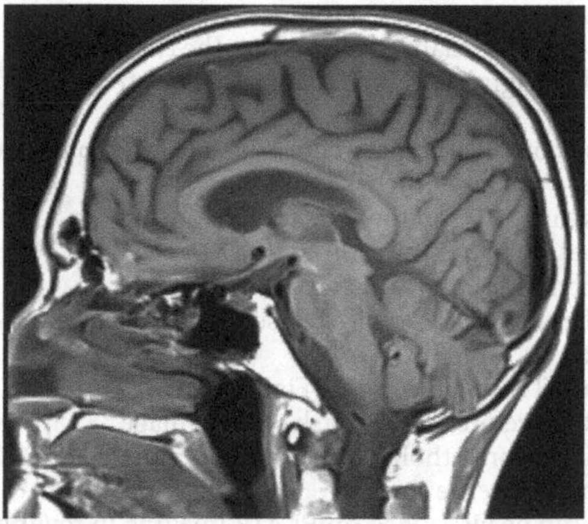

Figure 6.5 MRI; T1; sagittal view.

Source: Courtesy of Penn State Health Radiology Department.

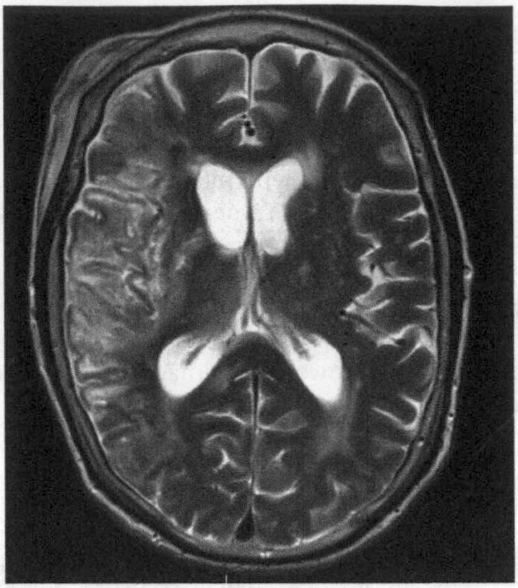

Figure 6.6 MRI; T2; axial view.

Source: Courtesy of Penn State Health Radiology Department.

- The most common MRI sequences used in stroke are diffusion weighted imaging (DWI), apparent diffusion coefficient (ADC), T2 fluid attenuated inversion recover (FLAIR), and susceptibility weighted imaging (SWI).
  - DWI
    - Produces images via movement or "diffusion" of water molecules (Brownian motion)
    - In stroke, ischemic tissue leads to swelling of cells and obstructed extracellular space, limiting movement of water
    - Produces a hyperintense lesion
    - Stroke can be visualized early from the time of onset
    - Reliable imaging to reveal acute ischemic stroke (Ermak, 2019)
  - ADC
    - Opposite of DWI in that acute ischemia is hypointense
    - Reaches peak hypointensity at around 4 days
    - Begins to then trend towards back to normal
    - Becomes isointense by around day 7 to 10
    - Will then be bright from this point forward
    - "Pseudonormalization" of ADC suggests subacute stroke (Ermak, 2019)
  - T2 FLAIR
    - Standard T2, fluid is bright (Figure 6.7)
    - FLAIR, therefore, CSF is dark on this image
    - This allows for pathology to be viewed more optimally as these show up as hyperintense (bright)
    - Stroke can be visualized on FLAIR imaging in roughly 6 hours from onset
    - Most common/useful imaging modality to evaluate for pathologies

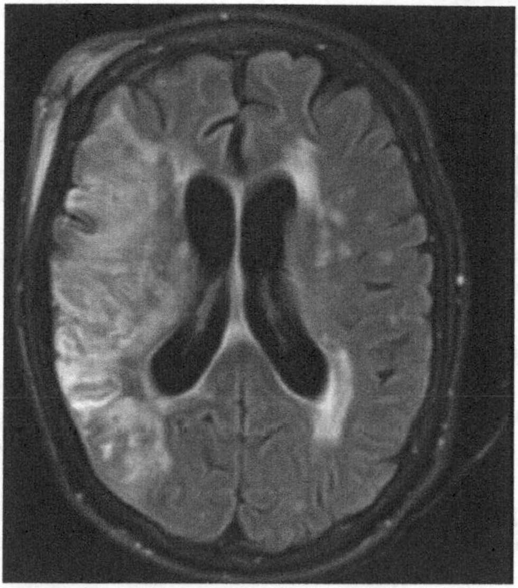

Figure 6.7 MRI; T2 FLAIR; axial view.

Source: Courtesy of Penn State Health Radiology Department.

FAST FACTS

Acute ischemic stroke is hyperintense on DWI, hypointense on ADC, and hyperintense on T2 imaging (if completed after roughly 6 hours from onset) and can help differentiate acute stroke from subacute.

- SWI
  - Images substances that are able to be magnetized (blood, iron, and calcium; Thamburaj, 2020)
  - Blood regardless of age will show signal dropout/hypointense
  - Some facilities may use T2* or gradient recalled echo (GRE) which are similar to SWI (Ermak, 2019)
  - Useful to evaluate patients for cerebral amyloid angiopathy and hypertensive microhemorrhages
  - Not indicated to obtain in acute ischemic stroke patients; however, if a prior MRI exists and SWI/GRE/T2* imaging was completed, may be helpful in risk stratification for thrombolytic therapy
- Hemorrhage evolves on MRI as blood products are broken down over time. The T1 images and T2 images will have differing appearances depending on the age of the hemorrhage and thus can be used in determining the age of hemorrhage.

MR Angiogram

- With or without gadolinium contrast
- Time of flight techniques (TOF) use the flow of blood within vessels to obtain images
- May overestimate degree of stenosis since, in severely stenotic states, flow is limited to a degree that is not detectable by TOF
- Less able to detect changes within the wall of the vessels and does not show calcifications as readily as CTA
- TOF images susceptible to motion artifact which can limit quality of images (Ermak, 2019)

Transthoracic Echocardiogram

- Useful to evaluate for cardioembolic sources including left ventricular thrombus, valvular abnormalities, atrial thrombus, and cardiac tumors
- Detection of PFO with bubble study through injection of agitated saline

Transesophageal Echocardiogram

- May better visualize the left atrial appendage for thrombus, the atrial septum for PFO, and also the aortic arch for sources of emboli

Carotid Doppler

- Only to be used as a confirmatory test
  - Limited to evaluate the common carotid and cervical internal carotid artery
  - Does not give information on the entire internal carotid, only the proximal and cervical internal carotid artery (petrous, cavernous, or clinoid carotid)
  - Does not give any information on intracranial circulation
- Provides data on degree of stenosis as well as plaque morphology
  - Ulceration, heterogeneity of plaque, and calcification

Transcranial Doppler

- **Emboli study:** may help distinguish active carotid disease or other active embolic disease
  - Unilateral embolic hits may signify a symptomatic/active carotid disease with emboli arising from proximal internal carotid artery
- **Stenosis study:** confirm stenosis intracranially, noninvasive technique to evaluate degree of stenosis as well as any changes in stenosis such as with vasospasm
  - Useful in monitoring for vasospasm in subarachnoid hemorrhage
  - Typically, would need a baseline study if monitoring stenoses over time and for changes
- **Bubble study:** injection of agitated saline to evaluate for right to left shunt (PFO or intrapulmonary shunt)

References

Albers, G. W., Marks, M. P., Kemp, S., Christensen, S., Tsai, J. P., Ortega-Gutierrez, S., McTaggart, R. A., Torbey, M. T., Kim-Tenser, M., Leslie-Mazwi, T., & Sarraj, A. (2018). Thrombectomy for stroke at 6 to 16 hours with selection by perfusion imaging. *New England Journal of Medicine*, *378*, 708–718.

Barber, P. A., Demchuk, A. M., & Zhang, J. (2000). Validity and reliability of a quantitative tomography score in predicting outcome of hyperacute stroke before thrombolytic therapy. *Lancet*, *355*, 1670–1674.

Brinjikji, W., Demchuk, A. M., Murad, M. H., Rabinstein, A. A., McDonald, R. J., McDonald, J. S., & Kallmes, D. F. (2017). Neurons over nephrons: Systematic review and meta-analysis of contrast induced nephropathy in patients with acute stroke. *Stroke*, *48*, 1862–1868.

Demeestere, J., Wouters, A., Christensen, S., Lemmens, R., & Lansberg, M. G. (2020). Review of perfusion imaging in acute ischemic stroke: From time to tissue. *Stroke*, *51*, 1017–1024.

Ermak, D. (2019). *Neuroimaging*. Penn State Health Milton S. Hershey Medical Center.

Ma, H., Campbell, B. C., Parsons, M. W., Churilov, L., Levi, C. R., Hsu, C., Kleinig, T. J., Wijeratne, T., Curtze, S., Dewey, H. M., & Miteff, F. (2019). Thrombolysis guided by perfusion imaging up to 9 hours after onset of stroke. *New England Journal of Medicine*, *380*, 1795–1803.

Powers, W. J., Rabinstein, A. A., Ackerson, T., Adeoye, O. M., Bambakidis, N. C., Becker, K., Biller, J., Brown, M., Demaerschalk, B. M., Hoh, B., & Jauch, E. C. (2018). Guidelines for the early management of patients with acute ischemic stroke. *Stroke*, *49*, e46–e110.

Thamburaj, K. (2020). *Susceptibility weighted imaging*. Penn State Health Milton S. Hershey Medical Center.

Vagal, A., Wintermark, M., Nael, K., Bivard, A., Parsons, M., Grossman, A. W., & Khatri, P. (2019). Automated CT perfusion imaging for acute ischemic stroke. *Neurology*, *93*, 888–898.

Wing, S., & Markus, H. (2018). Interpreting CT perfusion in stroke. *Practical Neurology*, *19*(2), 136–142. https://doi.org/10.1136/practneurol-2018-001917

7

SECTION IV: CLINICAL CARE

Emergency Care: Prehospital and in the Emergency Department

Alicia Richardson

Prehospital and emergency care for acute stroke have advanced rapidly over the last 30 years. Since the Food and Drug Administration (FDA) approval of IV tissue plasminogen activator (tPA) for acute ischemic stroke (AIS) in 1996 followed by several pivotal mechanical thrombectomy trials in 2015 and 2018, stroke care now has strong evidence-based practice to support hyperacute treatments in the ED. These hyperacute treatments place additional emphasis on prehospital staff and make them the first critical piece in stroke care. Prehospital staff are making difficult decisions based on routing plans in their region, trying to determine which hospital is most qualified to care for a particular stroke patient. Stroke identification tools are no longer enough. Prehospital staff are expected to additionally screen the patient using a large vessel occlusion (LVO) tool. Several LVO tools have been published in the last 10 years, with no tool showing superiority over another. However, prehospital staff are often requested to use an LVO tool to decide if a patient should be taken to the nearest acute stroke-ready or primary stroke center facility or if they perhaps need to be transferred to a thrombectomy-capable center or comprehensive stroke enter. In some cases, this may mean bypassing a stroke center even when they may be closer in proximity.

PREHOSPITAL

- Only approximately 50% to 60% of hospitalized stroke patients arrive at the hospital via emergency medical services (EMS; Adeoye et al., 2019). Community outreach activities should be focused on stroke symptom recognition and activation of 9-1-1 EMS systems, decreasing stroke onset to the ED arrival times, and increasing the timeliness of IV thrombolytic and thrombectomy (Powers et al., 2019).

- Public knowledge of stroke signs and risk factors in the United States remains poor. Blacks and Hispanics have been noted to have lower awareness than the general population, leading to longer delays in seeking care (Adeoye et al., 2019).
- Earlier ED arrival, quicker ED evaluation, faster door-to-needle (DTN) times, along with increased number of treated patients are some benefits of using EMS when experiencing stroke symptoms (Adeoye et al., 2019).

Benefits of Prehospital Notification by Emergency Medical Services

- Hospital resources can be initiated prior to the patient's arrival.
- Hospital team can be waiting for the patient's arrival.
- CT scanner can be available for immediate, rapid evaluation.
- Associated with increased likelihood of receiving thrombolysis, shorter door-to-imaging times, shorter DTN times, and shorter symptom onset-to-needle times (Adeoye et al., 2019)

Key Components of Prehospital Care

- Perform stroke screening tool. If positive, screen patient with an LVO tool.
- Establish last known well (LKW) time.
- Complete pre-hospital notification.
- Review past medical history (PMH) and current medication list.
- Review family/witness contact information.
- Obtain point-of-care (POC) blood glucose (rule out hypoglycemia as stroke mimic).
- Insert IV line, preferably two large bore.
- Stabilize stroke patient en route to ED.
- Keep nothing by mouth (NPO); do not treat hypertension and avoid dextrose-containing fluids.

Prehospital Assessments and Large Vessel Occlusion Tools

- Prehospital stroke screening tools are an important aspect of stroke care. The most common screening tools are as follows (Michel, 2017):
  - Cincinnati Prehospital Stroke Scale (CPSS)
  - Los Angeles Prehospital Stroke Screen (LAPSS)
  - Recognition of Stroke in the Emergency Room (ROSIER)
  - Face, Arm, Speech, Time (FAST)
- In 2016, a systematic review of the screening tools performance demonstrated that CPSS and FAST had similar sensitivity (range, 44%–95% for CPSS, 79%–97% for FAST), but both had poor specificity (range, 24%–79% for CPSS, 13%–88% for FAST; Powers et al., 2019). LAPSS had better specificity (range, 48%–97%) but poor sensitivity (range, 59%–91%). None of the tools accounted for false-negative cases and concluded that no strong recommendation can be made for one tool over another (Powers et al., 2019).
- The assessment on scene is recommended to be less than 15 minutes.
- Since thrombectomy has become standard of care, triage to a thrombectomy-capable stroke center is a critical decision for EMS personnel. Several LVO tools have since been developed and studied. The most common tools include the following:

  - VAN (Vision, Aphasia, Neglect)
  - RACE (Rapid Arterial oCclusion Evaluation Scale)
  - C-STAT (Cincinnati Stroke Triage Assessment Tool)
  - LAMS (Los Angeles Motor Scale)
  - PASS (Prehospital Acute Stroke Severity)
  - FAST-ED (Field Assessment Stroke Triage for Emergency Destination)
- Important characteristics of an LVO screening tool are as follows (Michel, 2017):
  - Simplicity, rapid to perform
  - Applicability to suspected AIS, including posterior circulation
  - High interrater reliability
  - High accuracy to identify strokes versus mimics
  - High accuracy to identify LVO versus non-LVO
  - Validated in external data sets and in the prehospital setting
  - Proven to improve patient outcomes

FAST FACTS

At this time, there is insufficient evidence to suggest one tool over another, and there are strengths and weaknesses to each tool (Adeoye et al., 2019). Some are limited by their complexity to rapidly perform which leads to poor integration into EMS practice, while others have poor sensitivity or specificity or have not been tested in the prehospital setting. To date, there is no head to head trial comparing the LVO tools.

- Regional or state protocols may indicate which LVO tool EMS personnel are to utilize.
- It is recommended that when there are several IV thrombolysis-capable centers in a geographical area, extra transportation times to reach a thrombectomy-capable center should be limited to no more than 15 minutes in an LVO tool positive patient (Adeoye et al., 2019). This topic is controversial, and further research is needed to establish travel time parameters for hospital bypass. The Mission Lifeline: Stroke Triage Algorithm for stroke severity, which was originally published in 2018, has been widely accepted.

MOBILE STROKE UNITS

In the last 10 years, mobile stroke units (MSUs) have emerged as an innovative way to improve the timeliness to stroke care. MSUs are CT-equipped ambulances staffed by a nurse, paramedic, and CT technician, with or without an onboard physician or advanced practice provider (APP); telemedicine is an alternative to having a provider on board.

- MSUs with the ability to perform a computed tomography angiography (CTA) facilitate confirmation of the presence of an LVO and transport to a thrombectomy-capable center.

- While costly and labor-intensive to implement and maintain, MSUs have been proven to be cost-effective when using disability-adjusted life years (Grotta et al., 2021).
- The BEST-MSU (Benefits of Stroke Treatment Delivered Using a Mobile Stroke Unit; compared with standard management by EMS) trial in 2021 demonstrated that MSU management of AIS in patients who were eligible to receive a thrombolytic resulted in less disability at 90 days and faster and more frequent thrombolytic treatment than standard EMS management (Grotta et al., 2021).
- Hemorrhagic stroke patients may be identified more quickly and therefore transported to an appropriate center (Adeoye et al., 2019).
- Lack of reimbursement from the government or third-party payers makes widespread implementation challenging and prohibitive (Adeoye et al., 2019).

EMERGENCY DEPARTMENT STROKE ALERT PROCESSES

- Organized structure and protocols within the ED for emergent evaluation of a suspected stroke patient are recommended (Powers et al., 2019).
- Designation of a "stroke team" in the ED provides clear role delineation when the stroke patient arrives. The stroke team is usually composed of an emergency medicine physician or APP, emergency nurse, pharmacist, CT technologist, and neurology physician or APP who responds to the notification of a stroke alert.
- Neurologic examination is most commonly performed by a member of the stroke team using a standardized tool such as the National Institutes of Health Stroke Scale (NIHSS). See Chapter 5 for more information on NIHSS.
- Historically, the first hour of stroke care was termed "the golden hour," with the goal of administering thrombolytic therapy within 60 minutes of hospital arrival. However, with the launch of the American Heart Association/American Stroke Association (AHA/ASA) Target Stroke Phase III initiative, the golden hour is now called "the golden half hour." Since many hospitals were meeting the goal of less than 60 minutes, the "golden half hour" (Table 7.1) encourages thrombolytic therapy within 30 minutes of hospital arrival.
- Prehospital personnel have likely already assisted ED staff by obtaining a POC blood glucose and inserting an IV. Some prehospital staff will have drawn additional labs and arrive with them. If not, emergency staff will obtain routine stroke labs.
- POC blood glucose and international normalized ratio (INR) for patients on warfarin are the only laboratory requirements prior to thrombolytic treatment, and obtaining labs should never delay administration of thrombolytics. The patient with an INR result >1.7 is not recommended for an IV thrombolytic, but could be a candidate for thrombectomy.

TABLE 7.1

30-Minute DTN Goal Time Intervals

Goal	Time
Door to physician	≤2.5 minutes
Door-to-stroke team	≤5 minutes
Door-to-CT/MRI initiation	≤15 minutes
Door-to-CT/MRI interpretation	≤25 minutes
DTN	≤30 minutes

DTN, door to needle.

Source: American Heart Association. (2018). *Target: Stroke phase III.* https://www.heart.org/en/professional/quality-improvement/target-stroke/introducing-target-stroke-phase-iii

FAST FACTS

While alteplase is the only FDA approved thrombolytic for AIS, tenecteplase has become the standard of care for many institutions as it was shown to be noninferior to alteplase in the AHA/ASA Ischemic Stroke Guidelines in 2019 (Powers et al., 2019). See Chapter 10 for more information on alteplase and tenecteplase.

Large Vessel Occlusion Evaluation

- In addition to evaluating a stroke patient for thrombolytic candidacy, the stroke team is also responsible for evaluating for LVO. If noted, and the center is thrombectomy-capable, the patient should be rapidly transported to the procedural area. (Thrombectomies are performed in a variety of locations depending on hospital structure; the neurointerventional radiology suite, cath lab, and operating rooms are common locations.) See Chapter 8 for more information on thrombectomy.
- If the center is not capable of performing a thrombectomy, an emergent interfacility transfer should be initiated.
- A quality metric to indicate timely transfers is a door-in-door-out (DIDO) time, with a goal of less than 90 minutes from the hospital ED "door in" (arrival) to hospital ED "door-out" (transfer).
- Best practices for improving DIDO times have been identified as (AHA, 2018):
  - Establishing the institutional goal for DIDO (example: less than 90 minutes DIDO for at least 50% of AIS patients)
  - Rapid administration of IV thrombolytics
  - Rapid initiation of transfer (examples: transfer agreements with automatic acceptance, prenotification to EMS with parallel workflows or EMS waiting for LVO diagnosis)
  - Participation in regional stroke care

- Use of telemedicine
- Rapid acquisition, interpretation, and transmission of neuroimaging
- Expedited transport handoff
- Mock stroke alerts
- Data collection, feedback, and quality improvement plans

- Thrombectomy-capable centers have the goals shown in Table 7.2 for door-to-device (DTD) times (AHA, 2018).
- For LVO patients arriving at thrombectomy-capable centers, processes allowing for the patient to bypass the ED and go straight to the procedural area decrease DTD time and increase the chance of better functional outcome.

HEMORRHAGIC STROKE IN THE EMERGENCY DEPARTMENT

- Intraparenchymal hemorrhage (IPH) and subarachnoid hemorrhage (SAH) patients are an important subset of stroke patients presenting to the ED, accounting for 12% of all stroke types. If an IPH or SAH is detected during the stroke, alert the CT head. The patient may undergo a CTA for further evaluation, as it could identify an aneurysm as the cause for the SAH or an arteriovenous malformation (AVM) as the cause for the IPH.

TABLE 7.2

Goals for DTD Times

Door to physician	≤5 minutes
Door-to-stroke team	≤10 minutes
Door-to-CT/MRI initiation	≤20 minutes
Door-to-CT/MRI interpretation	≤35 minutes
Door-to-neurointerventional team activation	≤40 minutes
DTN time	≤45 minutes
Door-to-patient arrival in neurointerventional suite	≤60 minutes
DTP	≤75 minutes
DTD	≤90 minutes

DTD, door to device; DTN, door to needle; DTP, door to puncture.

Source: American Heart Association. (2018). *Target: Stroke phase III*. https://www.heart.org/en/professional/quality-improvement/target-stroke/introducing-target-stroke-phase-iii

FAST FACTS

Presence of spot sign indicates the patient has active bleeding and hemorrhage expansion.

- If hemorrhage is identified, blood pressure (BP) management and reversal of coagulation become the main goals in the ED. Determining the need for transfer for neurosurgical services or higher level of care also occurs in parallel. The same DIDO described in Table 7.1 can be applied to hemorrhagic stroke transfers.
- IPH while on anticoagulation is associated with extremely high mortality and morbidity (Greenberg et al., 2022). It is important to identify which anticoagulant the patient was taking, so appropriate reversal can be initiated immediately, and typically prior to transfer (if warranted).
  Examples include:
  - Vitamin K antagonists (sarfarin)
  - Thrombin inhibitors (dabigatran)
  - Factor Xa inhibitors (rivaroxaban, apixaban)
- In patients with spontaneous IPH, high BP should be lowered using careful titration to ensure smooth and sustained control of BP; avoiding peaks to the systolic blood pressure (SBP) can improve functional outcomes (Greenberg et al., 2022).
- For a patient presenting with mild to moderate IPH, SBP between 150 and 220 mmHg, acute lowering to a target of 140 mmHg is safe and reasonable (Greenberg et al., 2022). For patients presenting with large or severe IPH or those requiring surgical decompression, the safety and efficacy of acute blood pressure lowering is not well established, and further research is needed (Greenberg et al., 2022).
- If acute lowering is indicated, initiating the treatment within 2 hours of IPH onset and reaching the target within 1 hour is associated with reduced risk of hematoma expansion and improved outcomes (Greenberg et al., 2022).

THROMBOLYTIC ADMINISTRATION

- Inclusion/exclusion criteria are reviewed by a member of the stroke team.
- The patient and/or family are informed of the risks/benefits with thrombolytic, and provide verbal consent to treatment.
- BP should be less than 185/110 before treatment.
- Frequent neurologic checks and vital signs ensure early detection of a change in patient status.
- Angioedema occurs in <1% of patients; protocols should be in place to manage angioedema and protect the patient's airway.
- Symptomatic intracerebral hemorrhage (sICH) rates postthrombolyic range between 2% and 6%, and therefore should be monitored postadministration. BP management postadministration is critical to decreasing the odds of having an sICH. If an sICH is suspected, immediately stop the infusion, if applicable, and obtain a noncontrast computerized tomography (NCCT).

FAST FACTS

If the patient is unable to verbalize consent and no family is present, remember that thrombolytics are standard of care for the treatment of an AIS and should be administered.

References

Adeoye, O., Nystrom, K., Yavagal, D., Luciano, J., Nogueria, R., Zorowitz, R., Khalessi, A., Bushnell, C., Barsan, W., Panagos, P., Alberts, M., Tiner, C., Schwamm, L., & Jauch, E. (2019). Recommendations for the establishment of stroke systems of care: A 2019 update. *Stroke*, *50*(7), e187–e210. https://doi.org/10.1161/STR.0000000000000173

AHA. (2018). *Target stroke phase III initiative.* https://www.heart.org/en/professional/quality-improvement/target-stroke/introducing-target-stroke-phase-iii

Greenberg, S., Ziai, W., Cordonnier, C., Dowlatshahi, D., Francis, B., Goldstein, J., Hemphill, C., Johnson, R., Keigher, K., Mack, W., Mocco, J., Newton, E., Ruff, I., Sansing, L., Schulman, S., Selim, M., Sheth, K., Sprigg, N., & Sunnerhagen, K. (2022). Guideline for the management of patients with spontaneous intracerebral hemorrhage: A guideline from the American Heart Association/American Stroke Association. *Stroke*, *53*, e282–e361. https://doi.org/10.1161/STR.0000000000000407

Grotta, J., Yamal, M., Parker, S., Rajan, S., Gonzales, N., Jones, W., Alexandrov, A., Navi, B., Nour, M., Spokoyny, I., Mackey, J., Persse, D., Jacob, A., Schimpf, B., Ackerson, K., Sherman, C., Lerario, M., Mir, S., Willey, J., … Bowry, R. (2021). Prospective, multicenter, controlled trial of mobile stroke units. *New England Journal of Medicine*, *385*, 11.

Michel, P. (2017). Prehospital scales for large vessel occlusion: Closing in on a moving target. *Stroke*, *48*, 247–249. https://doi.org/10.1161/STROKEAHA.116.015511

Powers, W., Rabinstein, A., Ackerson, T., Adeoye, O., Bambakidis, N., Becker, K., Biller, J., Brown, M., Demaerschalk, B., Hoh, B., Jauch, E., Kidwell, C., Leslie-Mazwi, T., Ovbiagele, B., Scott, P., Sheth, K., Southerland, A., Summers, D., & Tirschwell, D. (2019). Guidelines for the early management of patients with acute ischemic stroke: 2019 update to the 2018 guidelines for the early management of acute ischemic stroke. *Stroke*, *50*, e344–e418. https://doi.org/10.1161/STR.0000000000000211

8

Endovascular and Surgical Management of Stroke

Tina Resser and Daniel Wadden

Advances in open and endovascular neurosurgical techniques are changing stroke practice as we know it. This chapter briefly reviews acute endovascular interventions in ischemic stroke, as well as surgical management of carotid disease, ischemic, and hemorrhagic stroke.

ENDOVASCULAR THERAPY IN ISCHEMIC STROKE

Introduction

In patients presenting with acute ischemic stroke (AIS), up to 46% may be due to large vessel occlusions (LVO). AIS patients with ischemic penumbra and a LVO may benefit from endovascular therapy. This generally refers to mechanical thrombectomy (MT), or a mechanical removal of clot from the artery. Intra-arterial thrombolytic therapy may also be considered in select cases. While 10% to 17% of AIS patients may be eligible for endovascular treatment, only 3.1% undergo MT.

Thrombectomy Then and Now

Endovascular intervention began in the 1990s as a way to improve patient outcomes in patients who were not eligible for or did not benefit from alteplase. The Mechanical Embolus Removal in Cerebral Ischemia (MERCI) device was the first mechanical device for thrombectomy and was Food and Drug Administration (FDA) approved in 2004. Subsequent randomized control trials failed to demonstrate superiority over medical management, likely due to both patient selection criteria as well as time to recanalize using a "first generation" device. Intra-arterial therapy was not proven to be superior to IV alteplase during this time. Neuro-interventionalists turned to coronary technology and self-expanding stents off-label as an emergency rescue therapy.

The use of "stentrievers" was subsequently researched. Five trials (MR CLEAN, ESCAPE, REVASCAT, SWIFT PRIME, and EXTEND intracranial aneurysms [IA]) all demonstrated benefit. A subsequent meta-analysis of these trials, HERMES, demonstrated that the number needed to treat to improve three-month disability scores was one in 2.6. Improvement in endovascular technology subsequently included the growing field of aspiration catheters. These may be used instead of or as an adjunct device in the mechanical removal of clot. New large-bore aspiration catheters demonstrated superior recanalization rates but similar clinical outcomes to MT in trial.

Indications for Mechanical Thrombectomy

- Patients presenting 0 to 6 hours after symptom onset can be considered for both IV thrombolysis and MT. Evaluation for MT should ideally include noninvasive vessel imaging (CT angiography) to determine presence of LVO. Some providers/hospital systems may consider bringing a patient directly to the angiography suite for catheter angiography without CT angiogram to decrease door to needle time. For anterior circulation strokes, consideration for MT up to 24 hours post symptom onset may be appropriate when a patient meets criteria of the drug abuse warning network (DAWN) or DEFUSE 3 trials (see Chapter 17, Stroke Research and the Advanced Practice Provider). Strong consideration is given for MT in patients with LVO and National Institutes of Health Stroke Scale (NIHSS) >5; some endovascular providers will consider intervention with lower NIHSS based on significance of deficit observed. Trials are being completed to evaluate the efficacy of MT in patients with low NIHSS.
  - American Heart Association (AHA) guidelines recommend MT for patients that meet the following criteria:
    - Prestroke modified rankin scale (mRS) score of 0 to 1;
    - Causative occlusion of the internal carotid artery (ICA) or middle cerebral artery (MCA) segment 1 (M1);
    - Age (18 years or older);
    - NIHSS score of (greater than or equal to six); and
    - Treatment can be initiated (arterial puncture) within 6 hours of symptom onset.
  - AHA further suggests potential benefit of MT with stent retrievers in carefully selected patients with AIS when treatment can be initiated within 6 hours of symptom onset in patients with LVO in the M2 or M3 segment of the MCA.
  - MT utilizing stent retriever, direct aspiration, and/or intra-arterial fibrinolysis within 6 hours of symptoms are within AHA guidelines (Powers et al., 2019).
  - The goal of MT is to obtain Thrombolysis in Cerebral Infarction (TICI) 3 grade reperfusion as quickly as possible (Table 8.1).
- Greater than 6 hours from symptom onset, perfusion imaging (CT perfusion or medical representative [MR] perfusion) provides greater information on the core infarction size and penumbra size. Trials are being done to evaluate the efficacy of thrombectomy in patients with a large core

TABLE 8.1

Thrombolysis in Cerebral Infarction Score

TICI 0	No perfusion or antegrade flow beyond site of occlusion
TICI 1	Contrast passes the area of occlusion but fails to opacify the entire cerebral bed distal to the obstruction during angiographic run
TICI 2a	Partial (<50% of territory visualized) perfusion wherein the contrast passes the occlusion and opacifies the distal arterial bed but rate of entry or clearance from the bed is slower than noninvolved territories
TICI 2b	Partial (>50% of territory visualized) perfusion wherein the contrast passes the occlusion and opacifies the distal arterial bed but rate of entry or clearance from the bed is slower than noninvolved territories
TICI 2c	Near complete perfusion except for slow flow in a few distal cortical vessels or presence of small distal cortical emboli
TICI 3	Complete reperfusion with normal filling

Note: The TICI score is a grading scale for post thrombectomy to reflect the territory reperfused post clot retrieval (Spiotta et al., 2019).

TICI, thrombolysis in cerebral infarction.

on Alberta stroke program early CT (ASPECTS) or perfusion imaging (SELECT 2).

- Patients with prestroke (baseline) mRS of three or greater do poorly with MT. In patients with significant comorbidities (cancer, prior strokes, etc.) and poor baseline functioning, successful recanalization does not always lead to good outcomes.

POSTERIOR CIRCULATION STROKE CONSIDERATIONS

- Posterior fossa strokes are not well visualized on CT due to artifacts from bony structures in the cranial base, and early ischemic changes may be missed (Samaniego & Hasan, 2019).
- MRI with FLAIR and diffusion weighted imaging (DWI) sequences is ideal for evaluation of stroke burden in patients with posterior circulation LVO being considered for MT.
- The BASICS study showed diminishing benefit of MT with time from last known well (LKW) time, concluding consideration of MT if it can be accomplished within 6 hours. However, 23% to 35% of patients intervened after 6 hours still showed good outcomes, with 24% having good functional outcomes when MT occurred 12 to 24 hours from LKW (Samaniego & Hasan, 2019).

FAST FACTS

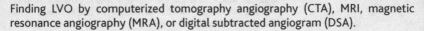

LVO definition:

- Anterior circulation (Fasen et al., 2020): occlusion of ICA and proximal M1 or M2 segments of the MCA
- Posterior circulation: occlusion of basilar artery and intracranial vertebral artery segments (Stib et al., 2020)
  See Chapter 3, Figures 3.11, 3.12, and 3.13.

FAST FACTS

Finding LVO by computerized tomography angiography (CTA), MRI, magnetic resonance angiography (MRA), or digital subtracted angiogram (DSA).

- Newer technologies (artificial intelligence [AI]) utilized to aid in detection of LVO are being employed to improve intervention time for patients with concern for LVO on noninvasive imaging. These tools have the ability to push images of CTAs to providers moments after a scan is completed where the AI suspects LVO.

ENDOVASCULAR TREATMENT OPTIONS

Patient Preparation

Once a patient is determined to be a candidate for thrombectomy, while the patient is brought to interventional suite, the interventionalist will determine the approach based on noninvasive imaging and target vessel. When possible, have updated lab work ready, including complete blood count (CBC), metabolic panel (specifically renal function), type, and screen. Update the patient's medical history and surgical history as knowing femoral stents, aortic stents/aneurysm, and femoral artery-popliteal artery bypass all help the proceduralist plan the safest and best route of access. Obtain informed consent per facility protocol.

Radial Versus Femoral Artery Access Approach

- Determine access site based on
  - Target vessel (left vs. right), ICA versus M1 versus M2, anterior versus posterior circulation
  - Anatomy: aortic arch (Type 1, 2, or 3, bovine), aberrant subclavian, radial artery (size, patent ulnar artery)
  - Guide catheter, intermediate catheter, microcatheter/microwire
    - Alternative systems coming out to market (Route 92 system)

Mechanical Aspiration

- Utilization of aspiration (suction) catheters via locking syringe or pump to remove clot from vessel

- 5fr (distal M1 and proximal M2), 6Fr, 7Fr, or 8Fr (ICA and proximal M1) aspiration catheters typically used
  - Sofia 5Fr and 6Fr (Microvention), React .071" (Medtronic) RED 62, 68, and 72 (Penumbra Inc.), Highpoint .070" and .088" (Route 92); other devices on market and available; utilization varies from facility to facility and proceduralist to proceduralist

Stentriever

- Wire-mounted stent (mesh tube) utilized to ensnare clot and open vessel
- Utilized as independent intervention or in combination with aspiration (Solumbra)
- Varying diameters and lengths of device chosen based on vessel size
- Solitaire (Medtronic), Embotrap (Cerenovus/J&J), Trevo (Stryker); other devices available; utilization varies from facility to facility and proceduralist to proceduralist

Other

- Intra-arterial thrombolytic instillation (tissue plasminogen activator [TPA] or tenecteplase [TNK])
  - Sometimes used in conjunction with thrombectomy

Complications of Thrombectomy

- Post-MT intracerebral hemorrhage (ICH)
  - Occurs in 4.4% of MT patients (Krishnan et al., 2021).
  - Caused by disruption of the blood–brain barrier (BBB) as a result of damage of the endothelium from MT technique and/or ischemic injury. These result in increased permeability of the tissue (Krishnan et al., 2021).
  - Early detection may be performed in interventional radiology (IR) suite utilizing flat panel detector CT head.
  - On post-angiogram, CT head (CTH) may see contrast versus hemorrhage; in these scenarios dual energy CTH can be performed to differentiate between hemorrhagic component and/or contrast.
  - Consider reversal of antithrombotic, fibrinolytics, and anticoagulant agents in setting of ICH.
  - European Cooperative Acute Stroke Study (ECASS) and Heidelberg Bleeding Classification both provide scoring for various postthrombolysis and post-MT ICH.
- Reocclusion of vessel
  - Occurs in 3% of MT patients (Krishnan et al., 2021)
  - Typically, within the first 48 hours postthrombectomy
  - May be caused by stenosis of the vessel, residual thrombus, and endothelial damage
  - Patients with suspicion of reocclusion of vessel should have emergent imaging completed to evaluate brain parenchyma and patency of cerebral vasculature. If core infarction has not significantly progressed and vessel is re-occluded, consideration for reperfusion attempt with MT is warranted.

- Post MT cerebral edema
  - Cerebral edema is a normal occurrence after ischemic injury to brain tissue. Monitoring for malignant edema is critical in management of the post-MT patient with LVO.
  - Edema begins around 6 hours postischemic event and typically peaks between three and five days postischemic event.
  - Please see Chapter 9, ICU Stroke Care, for acute management of cerebral edema.
  - Data shows that decompressive hemicraniectomy in patients >60 years of age results in increased morbidity and mortality (Krishnan et al., 2021).

Access Site Complications

- Hemorrhagic
  - Active bleeding from access site or hematoma formation may occur.
    - Management initially for both is manual compression until hemostasis/stopping of hematoma expansion.
    - Likely will need prolonged bedrest for femoral access patients.
    - Obtain arterial duplex US to assess for hematoma size and presence of pseudoaneurysm.
    - Retroperitoneal bleeding is also possible; intervention is dependent on patient's stability. This is potentially a life-threatening complication. Intervention ranges from monitoring to administration of blood products/pressor support to emergent surgical intervention.
- Occlusive
  - Occlusion of radial artery or femoral artery may occur.
    - Radial artery occlusion may be asymptomatic if ulnar collateral filling is sufficient.
    - Femoral artery occlusion due to clot formation, closure device impeding blood flow, or vessel dissection is an emergency and is likely to require vascular surgery intervention to manage.
  - Assessment of patient's distal pulses (dorsalis pedis, posterior tibial, popliteal, or distal radial [snuffbox]) prior to procedure will enable timely recognition of reduction/occlusion of arterial flow postarterial access for intervention.
  - Routine, frequent assessment of distal pulses by the RN and/or team providing care postarterial access should be part of the protocol for care post MT.

Anesthesia Considerations in Thrombectomy

General anesthesia (GA) versus conscious sedation (CS) during thrombectomy may be considered. Outcomes are mixed regarding outcome between the two choices in trial. CS can offer less hemodynamic instability and the ability to monitor the patient's neurologic exam, but aspiration and agitation are important risks. Consider GA in patients with difficult-to-control agitation, airway protection concerns, and clinical deterioration.

DECOMPRESSIVE SURGERY FOR MALIGNANT INTRACRANIAL EDEMA

Large strokes in the anterior or posterior fossa can be at risk for causing secondary injury via their mass effect. If large enough, they may progress to herniation, additional stroke, or death. Decompressive surgery refers to removal of part of the cranium to allow for the brain to swell out of its normally protected but confined space. This surgery may be considered for both ischemic and hemorrhagic strokes. For information on decompressive surgery for posterior fossa stroke, see the section Infratentorial Hemorrhage Evacuation later in this chapter.

Decompressive Hemicraniectomy in Ischemic Stroke

- May be considered in treatment of edema secondary to malignant MCA ischemic stroke
- Cerebral edema following stroke often develops after 24 to 48 hours.
- Reduces mortality and severe disability compared to medical management alone
- Young patients (<60 years) more likely to benefit
- Older adult patients (>60 years) may benefit but have much higher mortality or disability regardless of treatment.

Edema Identification

Development of cerebral edema is expected following acute stroke. Identifying *which strokes* are more likely to require subsequent medical management for edema and are at risk for surgical decompression is key. Close observation, management, and early neurosurgical consultation should be considered for the following (Dower et al., 2022):

- NIHSS ≥16 *and*
- Acute stroke size >50% of the MCA territory by imaging or >145 cm^3 volume of infarct on DWI sequence
- Age <60 years
- Hemodynamic stability
- Controlled coagulation
- Premorbid mRS 0 to 2 prior to acute stroke

FAST FACTS

Age >60 years, poor life expectancy >6 months prior to stroke (e.g., incurable metastatic malignancy), poor neurological baseline prior stroke, and high operative risk may exclude a patient from surgical candidacy. A discussion with the neurosurgical team in this patient group is helpful. Moreover, it is vital to discuss anticipated neurologic deficits and set realistic expectations with patient and family about stroke outcome, regardless of surgical candidacy.

PREOPERATIVE MANAGEMENT

- Airway, breathing, circulation
  - Monitor for and avoid aspiration, hypercapnia, hypoxemia.
  - Consider endotracheal intubation for Glasgow Coma Scale (GCS) less than 8.
- Medical management (see Chapter 9, ICU Stroke Care)
- Hourly neurological assessments with immediate surgical update for any decrease in level of consciousness, anisocoria, or worsening ipsilateral or contralateral limb weakness
- Frequent imaging at discretion of neuroscience teams to monitor for any progression in midline shift or mass effect
- Monitoring of coagulation and platelet studies
  - Aspirin is generally able to be continued through the perioperative period.
  - Additional antiplatelet, oral, or other anticoagulants may need to be adjusted or held at the discretion of the neurosurgical team.

OPERATIVE MANAGEMENT

- Perioperative antibiotics and antiepileptic therapy
- Incision shape may be large "T" (vertical incision anterior to ear meets midline incision from widow's peak posterior point near inion) or "question mark" (preauricular incision swoops over ear and posteriorly back near the inion before arching forward across midline to widow's peak)
- Large fragment of bone is excised, often >15 cm
- Bone may be sterilely packaged, preserved, and saved in operative suites for future replacement. Some institutions may choose creating a "pouch" in the patient's abdomen and temporarily implanting bone flap
- Dura is opened to allow bone to swell out
- Dural substitute is placed over exposed brain
- Skin incision is closed after meticulous control of any bleeding
- Drain may be used; cranial dressing applied

POSTOPERATIVE MANAGEMENT

- Perioperative antibiotics
- Postoperative CT for stability
- If postoperative CT demonstrates gross improvement in mass effect, osmotic therapy may be weaned within 24 hours.
- Surgical drain and dressing typically removed within 48 hours
- Hemicraniectomy precautions (see Table 8.2)
- Cranial suture removal 14 days after surgery

Complications of Hemicraniectomy

- Infection
- Bleeding
- Herniation of brain through skull defect

TABLE 8.2

Hemicraniectomy Precautions

Avoid patient lying on defect side.
Avoid tight straps across defect.
Fit helmet with patient; provide instructions to family for use.
Wear helmet when weight-bearing out of bed.

Note: Hemicraniectomy precautions refers to a number of safety parameters in the patient with an acquired bone flap defect to prevent pressure being placed directly on the brain.

- Postoperative hygroma or hematoma
- External compressive injury
- Degradation of bone flap
- Sinking skin flap syndrome
  - Development of neurologic symptoms due to concave "sunken" scalp at side of bony defect

Bone flap replacement, or "cranioplasty" can be scheduled once the swelling has decreased to the point that the bone can be safely reattached. In most cases, this occurs after eight weeks.

SURGICAL CONSIDERATIONS IN CAROTID STENOSIS

Asymptomatic Carotid Stenosis

- Best medical management and risk factor reduction is the primary goal for any patient with asymptomatic carotid stenosis.
- Surgical benefit for asymptomatic disease is controversial.
- Presence of clinically "silent" ipsilateral stroke or prior contralateral stroke or transient ischemic attack (TIA) may lead the surgeon to recommend treatment of asymptomatic carotid stenosis.
- Certain carotid imaging characteristics may increase a patient's risk of stroke and deem the stenosis unstable or at risk, leading to a decision for treatment (see Table 8.3).

Symptomatic Carotid Stenosis

- Defined as *symptomatic* when stenosis is the cause of a patient's amaurosis fugax, TIA, or ischemic stroke.
- Best medical management should be practiced.
- If carotid stenosis is the suspected cause of stroke, carotid surgical team (e.g., neurosurgery or vascular surgery) should be consulted for consideration of carotid revascularization.
- To reduce risk, carotid treatment following diagnosed symptomatic carotid stenosis is preferred within 14 days following a patient's admission for stroke (Abbott et al., 2015).

TABLE 8.3

Imaging Findings Associated With "At Risk" Asymptomatic Carotid Disease

Imaging finding	Modality
Impaired cerebral vascular reserve	TCD
Increased juxtaluminal black (hypoechogenic area)[a]	CUS, CTA, MRA, DSA
Intraplaque hemorrhage	CUS, CTA, MRA, DSA
Ipsilateral silent infarction	MRI, CT
Large plaque echolucency	CUS, CTA, MRA, DSA
Microemboli detected	TCD
Plaque ulceration	CUS, CTA, MRA, DSA
Stenosis progresses >20%	CTA, MRA, CUS, DSA

[a]Juxtaluminal black refers to fresh thrombus along the lumen without overlying fibrous cap.
CTA, computerized tomography angiography; CUS, carotid ultrasound; DSA, digital subtracted angiogram; MRA, magnetic resonance angiography; TCD, transcranial Doppler.

Treatment Options

Treatment of carotid stenosis includes carotid endarterectomy (CEA), carotid artery stenting (CAS), or transcarotid artery revascularization (TCAR; Kim et al., 2022). Anesthesia has a vital role in careful blood pressure management (Mohammaden et al., 2022).

- **CEA:** A surgical incision is made in the neck (parallel and posterior to the sternocleidomastoid muscle), platysma excised, and tissue carefully dissected until the ipsilateral carotid bifurcation is exposed. Prior to clamping of the common carotid, internal carotid, and external carotid arteries, anesthesia administers IV heparin and raises the patient's blood pressure. The arteries are then clamped, and the surgeon performs an arteriotomy with plaque excised. After the plaque is removed, the incision is closed and back bled to remove air and debris. The clamps are then removed. A surgical drain is often placed, and incision closed.
- **CAS:** The patient should be therapeutic on dual antiplatelet (see Table 8.4) medications prior to the procedure. Radial or femoral artery access is obtained once therapeutic; the procedure is performed in

FAST FACTS

Patients with prior neck radiation, anatomic considerations like high carotid bifurcation, high cardiovascular risk for CEA, or age >80 years may be better candidates for CAS or TCAR.

TABLE 8.4

Antiplatelet Medications Prescribed in Extracranial and Intracranial Stents

Medication	Half-Life	Loading Dose	Maintenance Dose
Aspirin Cyclooxygenase-1 inhibitor	30 minutes	650 mg oral/ feeding tube or rectal	81–325 mg/d oral/feeding tube or rectal
Clopidogrel P2Y12 inhibitor	7 hours	300 mg–600 mg oral/feeding tube	75 mg/d oral/feeding tube
Prasrugrel P2Y12 inhibitor	7 hours	20 mg–30 mg oral/ feeding tube	5 mg/d for weight <60 kg oral/ feeding tube 10 mg/d for weight >60 kg oral/feeding tube
Ticagrelor P2Y12 inhibitor	7 hours	180 mg oral/ feeding tube	90 mg/BID oral/feeding tube Use with 81 mg/d aspirin dose
Cangrelor[a] P2Y12 inhibitor	6 minutes	30 mcg IV bolus	4 mcg/kg/min IV Should be transitioned to oral P2Y12 inhibitor when feasible

Note: Some interventionalists will request lab work testing to confirm the patient is therapeutic on their dual antiplatelet medication. A platelet reactivity test (PRU) or aspirin/clopidogrel resistance panel may be ordered. Check to learn which test is available at the institution.

[a]Cangrelor is not usually prescribed in elective carotid stenting procedures but may be initiated if unplanned or emergent stenting occurs.

BID, bis in die.

the angiography suite. A guide catheter is advanced to the ipsilateral common carotid artery (CCA). A smaller micro catheter is advanced into the ICA past the area of narrowing and a distal embolic protection device deployed. A stent is then advanced over the microcatheter across the area of stenosis. Once properly positioned, it is deployed. The stent delivery wire is subsequently removed, and a balloon wire is advanced and carefully inflated temporarily across the stenosis, deflated, and removed. Imaging is repeated to confirm the stent is in good position, the stenosis is treated, and the carotid and cranial circulation is patent.

- **TCAR (Silk Road Medical Inc., Sunnyvale, CA)**: Patients should be therapeutic on dual antiplatelet medications prior to starting this procedure. This hybrid open/angiographic procedure involves both surgical dissection and stenting. The femoral vein is first accessed via catheterization. A small incision is then made in the neck to expose and secure the CCA. A sheath is placed in the CCA and secured. The sheath is then connected to a flow controller and subsequently attached to the femoral vein catheter. This adjustable flow reversal prevents distal emboli. While in flow reversal, a catheter is introduced via the common carotid sheath, crossing the area of stenosis. A balloon is inflated into the internal carotid artery and stent subsequently deployed. The catheters are then removed and arteriotomy closed.

POSTCAROTID CARE

- Regardless of procedure type, all patients should have a postoperative carotid ultrasound to rule out dissection.
- Vital signs should be carefully monitored. Any carotid manipulation can result in transient hypotension or bradycardia which may need treatment (usually self-remitting; Resser & Strayer, 2019).
- Avoid hypertension which can place patient at risk for reperfusion injury.
- CEA and TCAR should have perioperative antibiotics. Surgical drains, if placed, are typically removed the day after surgery.
- CEA patients should be continued on postoperative aspirin. CAS and TCAR patients should be counseled on the importance of dual antiplatelet compliance.
- Most patients are discharged home the next day.

Potential Complications

- Bleeding
- Infection
- Stroke
- Cerebral reperfusion syndrome
- Arterial dissection
- Cranial nerve injury
- Restenosis

INTRACEREBRAL HEMORRHAGE

Surgical treatment in ICH is a complicated discussion. In general, there are two categories of surgical consideration in patients admitted with ICH:

- Surgery to evacuate ICH
- Surgery to treat cause of ICH

Surgery to Evacuate Intracerebral Hemorrhage

The theoretical benefits to surgical evacuation of hemorrhage include the following:

- Improve outcome and reduce mortality by reducing direct injury to neural tissue
- Improve morbidity and reduce mortality by reducing secondary neural injury and cerebral edema following initial hemorrhage
- Prevent hematoma expansion
- Obtain pathology

Historical multicenter randomized trials have failed to find absolute improvement in outcome when evaluating open craniotomy with traditional surgical resection of supratentorial hemorrhage (bleeding in the cerebral cortex). As ICH is associated with the highest morbidity and mortality of all stroke subtypes, a continued interest in modern approaches to surgical evacuation have reinvigorated the interest in novel, minimally invasive surgical (MIS) approaches to evacuate hemorrhage. The largest recent randomized control to date, minimally invasive surgery with thrombolysis in intracerebral hemorrhage evacuation (MISTIE) III, improved mortality but did not improve functional outcome when comparing the treatment group to the control group. However, secondary analysis did demonstrate improvement in patient outcome who had a larger percentage of hemorrhage evacuated. As of the writing of this chapter, another randomized control trial using a minimally invasive device (ENRICH trial) has completed its trial and is due for a 2023 publication of results. Interested readers may research this trial as its results may alter future recommendations for surgical evacuation in hemorrhagic stroke.

SUMMARY OF 2022 GUIDELINES FOR HEMATOMA EVACUATION OF INTRACEREBRAL HEMORRHAGE

- Supratentorial hemorrhage >20 to 30 mL with GCS in five to 12 range, minimally invasive evacuation may be helpful to reduce mortality (Level 2A)
- Supratentorial hemorrhage >20 to 30 mL with GCS in five to 12 range, minimal invasive evacuation can be considered over conventional craniotomy to improve functional outcome (Level 2b)
- The effectiveness of minimally invasive hematoma evacuation for supratentorial hemorrhage >20 to 30 mL with GCS five to 12 is uncertain (Greenberg et al., 2022).

MINIMALLY INVASIVE SURGICAL HEMATOMA EVACUATION

The general principles of novel MIS techniques include careful patient selection, intraoperative stereotactic imaging, and minimally invasive or disruptive equipment (Musa et al., 2022). Several devices have been FDA approved for use. Techniques vary with some utilizing a small "mini" craniotomy with endoscopic evacuation or a large burr hole craniectomy device-guided aspiration. Neurosurgery should be consulted for all patients admitted with acute ICH to be evaluated for cause of bleed and need for surgical treatment.

Factors Favorable to Surgical Evacuation

- Age 18 to 80 years
- ICH volume >20 to 80 mL
- Presentation from LKW to treatment within 24 hours
- Lobar or anterior basal ganglia location of hemorrhage
- Mild to moderate clinical injury based on exam, GCS five to 14, and NIHSS score ≥6
- Premorbid modified Rankin score 0 to 1
- Absence of secondary lesion causing bleed, such as aneurysm, vascular malformation, or tumor
- Normalized coagulation

Factors Which May Exclude Candidacy for Evacuation

- Ruptured vascular malformation, aneurysm, hemorrhagic mass, prior ICH, or other vasculopathy

- Extensor posturing or fixed bilateral dilated nonreactive pupils
- Primary thalamic ICH
- Extensive intraventricular hemorrhage >50% of either lateral ventricle
- Brainstem location of hemorrhage
- Uncorrected coagulopathy or clotting disorder
- Thrombocytopenia (platelet <75,000 k/uL) or elevated INR >1.4 after correction
- Inability to correct anticoagulation
- Requirement that patient is on anticoagulation ≤5 days from initial hemorrhage
- Active gastrointestinal (GI), genitourinary (GU), retroperitoneal, or respiratory bleeding
- End-stage kidney or liver disease
- Mechanical heart valve
- Pregnancy
- Absence of reasonable expectation of recovery

Preoperative Management

- Blood pressure control
- Optimized medical therapy for cerebral edema (if indicated)
- Reversal of anticoagulants (see Chapter 10, Critical Care Pharmacology)
- Adequate platelets and stable coagulation factors
- Arterial line and Foley catheter placed
- Central line or large-bore peripheral IV access maintained

Perioperative Management

- The patient is positioned and placed under GA.
- Perioperative antibiotics and antiepileptics are prescribed.
- Neuronavigation equipment is set up and surgical trajectory is planned.
- The planned entry site is prepped.
- Incision is made and cranium opened via either burr hole or small craniotomy (depending on device used). Dura mater is subsequently opened before proceeding.
- MIS techniques:
  - Aspiration and thrombolysis: After burr hole is placed and dura opened, an aspiration catheter is advanced to the clot via imaging guidance. Gentle, single aspiration is applied and results removed. Infusion of thrombolytic agent then slowly infuses and drainage catheter is left in the hemorrhage bed so the clot can dissolve and passively drain out over the ensuing days prior to catheter removal.
  - Endoport evacuation: A small craniotomy is made and dura opened. Endoport device is advanced to clot using stereotactic imaging guidance. Inner obturator of the endoport is removed and the outer sheath is left in place. Surgeon then irrigates and removes the clot. At completion of evacuation, dura is closed and craniotomy bone defect is secured.

- Endoscopic evacuation: A small craniotomy or craniectomy is created, dura opened, and endoscope is advanced under stereotactic imaging guidance to clot. The hematoma is carefully suctioned out.
- Endoscopic endoport evacuation: A craniectomy is made and dura opened. The device is advanced to clot using stereotactic imaging guidance. When the clot is reached, the inner obturator is removed, and the outer sheath is left in place. The clot is then removed.

Postoperative Management

- Antibiotics and antiepileptics
- Postoperative CT brain
- Local wound management

Complications of Surgical Treatment of Intracerebral Hemorrhage

- Bleeding
- Infection
- Stroke
- Inadequate evacuation of hemorrhage
- Cerebral edema
- Seizure

Infratentorial Hemorrhage Evacuation

The indications and contraindications for resection of cerebellar hemorrhage are clearer. A patient with small cerebellar hemorrhage and GCS 14 to 15 should be monitored carefully for expansion or edema development. Conversely, ICH patients without brainstem reflexes and who are quadriplegic which do not improve after emergent osmotic therapy will likely not benefit from emergent surgical decompression. Spontaneous brainstem hemorrhage is not proven to benefit from surgical evacuation.

Surgery should be urgently considered for:

- Patients with GCS ≤ 13
- Cerebellar hematoma ≥4 cm, hydrocephalus, or brainstem compression
- Decompressive suboccipital craniectomy (SOC): This is a removal of the posterior fossa skull, with or without resection of hematoma. Decompressive SOC is also used to decompress in the event of cerebellar edema due to cerebellar ischemic stroke.
- Some cases have been reported of image-guided, minimally invasive evacuation of hematoma
  - Typically noted in smaller cases without malignant edema or herniation

Preoperative Management of Surgery for Infratentorial Hemorrhage

- Blood pressure control
- Optimized medical therapy for cerebellar edema
- Adequate platelets and stable coagulation factors

Perioperative Management of Suboccipital Craniectomy

The patient is positioned in a prone or lateral oblique position. Perioperative antibiotics are initiated. Once a sterile field is finalized, a midline longitudinal incision is made and subcutaneous tissue dissected, exposing occiput to the second cerebral vertebrae (C2). A craniotomy is created, and bone is carefully removed. A C1 laminectomy is often also performed to create a larger decompression. The dura is then opened. In the case of hemorrhage, the surgeon may choose to dissect the cerebellum at this point and evacuate the hematoma. Once the hematoma is evacuated, dural substitute is laid on the exposed cerebellum, and the fascia and skin are then closed. If an external ventricular drain is not already in place, one is typically placed prior to the patient returning to intensive care.

Postoperative Management of Surgery for Suboccipital Craniectomy

- Perioperative antibiotics
- Postoperative CT brain
- If brainstem compression or fourth ventricular effacement is noted on the postoperative image, continued osmotic therapy should be considered.
- External ventricular drain management
- Wound management and SOC precautions (see Table 8.5)

Complications of Suboccipital Craniectomy

- Infection
- Bleeding
- Pseudomeningocele (abnormal collection of cerebrospinal fluid protruding through skull defect)
- Ischemic stroke

Surgical Management of Underlying Causes of Intracerebral Hemorrhage

While most cases of hemorrhagic stroke are spontaneous and often due to hypertension, secondary causes may exist. In these cases, surgical treatment of cause may be necessary to reduce risk of bleeding and improve patient's outcome. Some secondary lesions include:

- Intracranial aneurysm
- Arteriovenous malformations (AVM) and dural arteriovenous fistula (dAVF)

TABLE 8.5

Suboccipital Craniectomy Precautions

Avoid tight straps across defect.
Helmet is not needed.
Avoid rubbing or friction across incision.

Note: Suboccipital craniectomy precautions refers to a number of safety parameters in the patient with an acquired posterior fossa bone flap defect.

- Cavernous malformations
- Tumors
- Infections

Detailed history and physical can help determine if a patient has risk factors for a secondary cause of hemorrhage. Young patients (<60 years of age), those with normotension at baseline, or imaging or vascular imaging that raises suspicion for secondary cause of hemorrhage should have further workup and neurosurgical consultation.

SURGICAL PLANNING FOR SECONDARY CAUSES OF INTRACEREBRAL HEMORRHAGE

When a secondary cause of hemorrhage is identified, the decision for surgery must account for two factors:

- Whether the causative lesion should be resected immediately to prevent further injury
- Whether the size of the hemorrhage is causing or will cause secondary injury and should be managed via open surgery

Aneurysm

- Ruptured aneurysms which cause ICH will always need early treatment to secure (Figure 8.1).
- May be secured with or without hemorrhage evacuation, depending on size and location of each.
- May be secured via open or endovascular methods.

Arteriovenous Malformation

- Rupture may not necessarily need urgent AVM treatment.
- Hemorrhage evacuation can often be timed with AVM resection if open treatment is considered.
- Ruptured AVM should be recommended for treatment, whether open surgical, endovascular, or via radiation. This decision is based on AVM characteristics, surgical opinion, and patient choice.
- dAVF is a type of malformation. If one bleeds, it should be treated via open or endovascular disconnection.

Cerebral Cavernous Malformation

- Cerebral cavernous malformations (CCM, also named cavernous angiomas or cavernomas) are low-flow vascular lesions comprised of thin, lobulated sinusoidal channels.
- They often do not need surgical treatment if they bleed and are often low risk for rebleeding. However, rebleeding CCMs, or those in the brainstem, may require surgical resection if found.

Tumor

- Hemorrhagic tumors may be metastatic or a primary brain malignancy. Benign brain tumors, such as hemangioblastomas, may also present with hemorrhage. Evaluation should include additional diagnostic imaging to

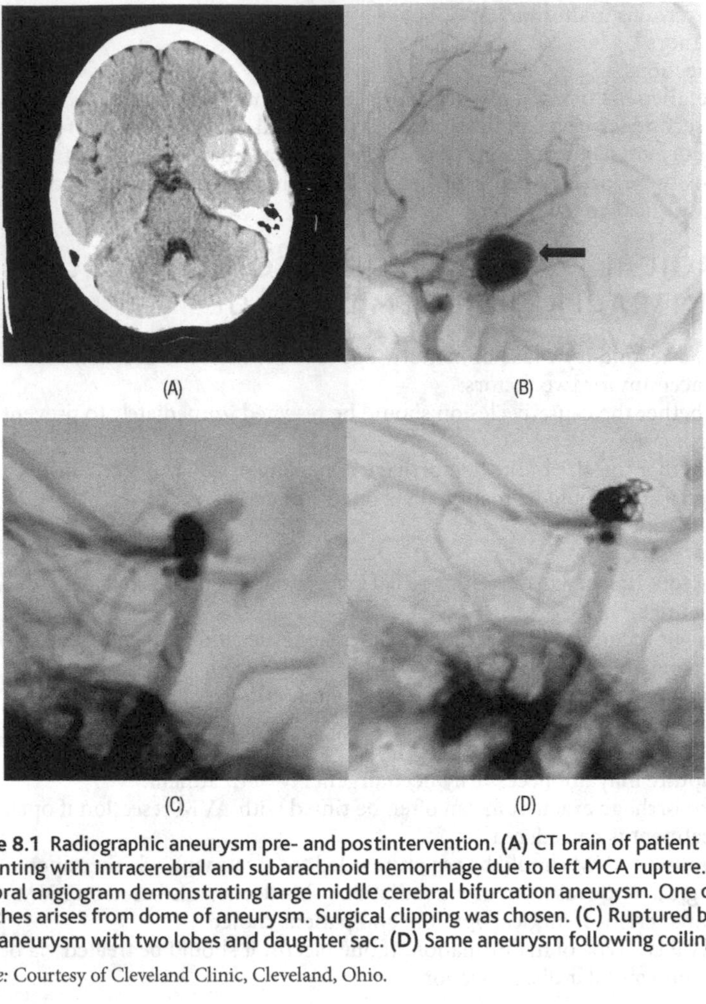

Figure 8.1 Radiographic aneurysm pre- and postintervention. **(A)** CT brain of patient presenting with intracerebral and subarachnoid hemorrhage due to left MCA rupture. **(B)** Cerebral angiogram demonstrating large middle cerebral bifurcation aneurysm. One of branches arises from dome of aneurysm. Surgical clipping was chosen. **(C)** Ruptured basilar apex aneurysm with two lobes and daughter sac. **(D)** Same aneurysm following coiling.

Source: Courtesy of Cleveland Clinic, Cleveland, Ohio.

determine if tumor is the expected cause, whether it is benign or malignant, and whether it is primary or metastatic malignancy. Surgical resection of the tumor and hemorrhage may help yield pathology (if one is not known). Adjunct consultations to medical and radiation oncology should be pursued once pathology is obtained.

Infection

- Patients with meningitis or encephalitis may develop ICH, or infection may present as a complication such as mycotic aneurysm. With the exception of mycotic aneurysm, other causes of infectious ICH are uncommon and do not routinely require neurosurgical treatment.

Surgical Management in Aneurysmal Subarachnoid Hemorrhage

Early treatment of ruptured IA treatment is essential to help prevent rebleeding. Rerupture is associated with higher morbidity and mortality. Following vessel imaging and aneurysm location, size, and morphology, treatment can be decided. See Chapter 9, ICU Stroke Care, for further care regarding detailed medical management of ruptured IA. Various treatment options can be reviewed in Table 8.6.

Care After Aneurysm Securement

- Open vascular treatment, such as clipping or bypass, will require perioperative antibiotics, as well as antiepileptic medications to prevent seizure after craniotomy.

TABLE 8.6

Methods of Intracranial Aneurysm Treatment

Aneurysm Securement	Open or Endovascular	Technical Notes
Coiling	Endovascular	Most commonly used securement for ruptured aneurysms. Involves catheter placement into aneurysm, followed by detachable coils strategically placed in aneurysm until aneurysm no longer fills. May require temporary balloon inflation or stent placement to "scaffold" coils in aneurysm and prevent coil protrusion in parent artery. If stents placed, patient must be on dual antiplatelet medications.
Flow Diversion	Endovascular	Class includes flow diverter stents whose design reduces porosity and reduces flow into/out of aneurysm, creating stasis in aneurysm and thrombus. Dual antiplatelet medication is needed to prevent in-stent thrombus. Intrasaccular FD are specially shaped and placed in body of aneurysm to create stasis of flow. Aspirin is often continued after the procedure.
Liquid embolic agents	Endovascular	Primarily utilized in distal aneurysms (e.g., mycotic). Onyx (Medtronic, Minneapolis, Minnesota) is a viscous embolic system that can be infused to occlude distal aneurysms unreached by traditional catheter systems.
Clipping	Open	Traditional craniotomy with surgical dissection and microsurgical clipping at the neck of an aneurysm. Can be helpful in aneurysms not easily amenable by endovascular techniques, or when hemorrhage evacuation or treatment also necessitates open surgical treatment.
Bypass	Open	Rarely used, generally utilized for giant aneurysms not amenable to other options. Craniotomy is performed and surgical bypass (either through local or grafted vessels) is performed to maintain blood flow to brain prior to aneurysm trapping and securement.

FD, flow diversion; MN, maternal newborn.

- The vast majority of open treatments include intraoperative angiography. Monitor vital signs, catheterization access site, and distal pulses for complications.
- Verify need and duration of any antiplatelet medications needed following endovascular treatment.

Complications of Aneurysm Treatment

- Bleeding
- Infection
- Stroke
- Arterial dissection
- Vasospasm
- Seizure
- Aneurysm recurrence
- Angiogram site complications such as vessel injury, bleeding, pseudoaneurysm

References

Abbott, A., Paraskevas, K. I., Kakkos, S. K., Golledge, J., Eckstein, H. H., Diaz-Sandoval, L. J., Cao, L., Fu, Q., Wijeratne, T., Leung, T. W., Montero-Baker, M., Lee, B. C., Pircher, S., Bosch, M., Dennekamp, M., & Ringleb, P. (2015). Systematic review of guidelines for the management of asymptomatic and symptomatic carotid stenosis. *Stroke*, *46*, 3288–3301.

Dower, A., Mulcahy, M., Maharaj, M., Chen, H., Lim, C. E. D., Li, Y., & Sheridan, M. (2022). Surgical decompression for malignant cerebral oedema after ischaemic stroke. *Cochrane Database of Systematic Reviews*, *2022*(11), 1–50.

Fasen, B. A. C. M., Heijboer, R. J. J., Hulsmans, F.-J. H., & Kwee, R. M. (2020, April). CT angiography in evaluating large vessel occlusion in acute anterior circulation ischemic stroke: Factors associated with diagnostic error in clinical practice. *American Journal of Neuroradiology*, *41*, 607–611.

Greenberg, S. M., Ziai, W. C., Cordonnier, C., Dowlatshahi, D., Francis, B., Goldstein, J. N., Hemphill III, J. C., Johnson, R., Keigher, K. M., Mack, W. J., Mocco, J., Newton, E. J., Ruff, I. M., Sansing, L. H., Schulman, S., Selim, M. H., Sheth, K. N., Sprigg, N., Sunnerhagen, K. S., & on behalf of the American Heart Association/American Stroke Association. (2022). 2022 guideline for the management of patients with spontaneous intracerebral hemorrhage: A guideline from the American Heart Association/American Stroke Association. *Stroke*, *53*, e282–e361. https://doi.org/10.1161/STR.0000000000000407

Kim, H. W., Regenhardt, R. W., D'Amato, S. A., Nahhas, M. I., Dmytriw, A. A., Hirsch, J. A., Silverman, S. B., & Martinez-Gutierrez, J. C. (2022). Asymptomatic carotid artery stenosis: A summary of current state of evidence for revascularization and emerging high-risk features. *Journal of Neurointerventional Surgery*, 1–8.

Krishnan, R., Mays, W., & Elijovich, L. (2021). Complications of mechanical thrombectomy in acute ischemic stroke. *Neurology*, *97*, S115–S125. https://doi.org/10.1212/WNL.0000000000012803

Mohammaden, M. H., Haussen, D. C., Al-Bayeti, A. R., Hassan, A. E., Tekle, W., Fifi, J. T., Matsoukas, S., Kuybu, O., Gross, B. A., Lang, M., Narayanan, S., Cortez, G. M., Hanel, R. A., Aghaebrahim, A., Sauvageau, E., Farooqui, M., Ortega-Gutierrez, S., Zevallos, C. B., Galecio-Castillo, M., & Nogueira, R. G. (2022). General anesthesia vs procedural sedation for failed neurothrombectomy undergoing rescue stenting: Intention to treat analysis. *Journal of Neurointerventional Surgery*, 1–8.

Musa, M. J., Carpenter, A. B., Kellner, C., Sigounas, D., Godage, I., Sengupta, S., Oluigbo, C., Cleary, K., & Chen, Y. (2022). Minimally invasive intracerebral hemorrhage evacuation: A review. *Annals of Biomedical Engineering, 50*(4), 365–386.

Powers, W. J., Rabinstein, A. A., Ackerson, T., Adeoye, O. M., Bambakidis, N. C., Becker, K., Biller, J., Brown, M., Demaerschalk, B. M., Hoh, B., Jauch, E. C., Kidwell, C. S., Leslie-Mazwi, T. M., Ovbiagele, B., Scott, P. A., Sheth, K. N., Southerland, A. M., Summers, D. V., & Tirschwell, D. L. (2019). Guidelines for the early management of patients with acute ischemic stroke: 2019 update to the 2018 guidelines for the early management of acute ischemic stroke: A guideline for health professionals from the American Heart Association/American Stroke Association. *Stroke, 50*(12), e344–e418.

Resser, T. S., & Strayer, A. L. (2019). Intracranial aneurysms. In J. V. Hickey & A. L. Strayer (Eds.), *The clinical practice of neurological and neurosurgical nursing* (8th ed., pp. 572–601). Wolters Kluwer.

Samaniego, E. A., & Hasan, D. (2019). *Acute stroke management in the Era of thrombectomy.* Springer.

Spiotta, A. M., Fiorella, D., Arthur, A. S., Frei, D., Turk, A. S., & Hirsch, J. A. (2019, March). The semiotics of distal thrombectomy: Towards a TICI score for the target vessel. *Journal of NeuroInterventional Surgery, 11*(3), 213–214.

Stib, M. T., Vasquez, J., Dong, M. P., Kim, Y. H., Subzwari, S. S., Triedman, H. J., Wang, A., Wang, H. L. C., Yao, A. D., Jayaraman, M., Boxerman, J. L., Eickhoff, C., Cetintemel, U., Baird, G. L., & McTaggart, R. A. (2020). Detecting large vessel occlusion at multiphase CT angiography by using a deep convolutional neural network. *Radiology, 297,* 640–649.

9

ICU Stroke Care

Kimberly Ichrist

There are guidelines and recommendations for the critical management of ischemic stroke, hemorrhagic stroke, and subarachnoid hemorrhage from the American Heart Association, the American Stroke Association, and the Neurocritical Care Society. However, guidelines do not specifically advise the admission process of a patient into the ICU. Each patient should have individualized care and evaluate the severity of the stroke such as location, size, deficits, edema and/or mass effect, compromise of vital functions, and comorbidities to provide optimal critical care management.

ISCHEMIC STROKE

Blood Pressure Management

Blood pressure management is an important aspect of stroke care. Despite hypertension being associated with stroke risk, initial care of the patient with ischemic stroke allows permissive hypertension to ensure adequate cerebral perfusion. Similarly, in patients with hemorrhagic transformation, blood pressure goals are lowered to prevent hematoma expansion. Recommended blood pressure targets are presented in Table 9.1.

TABLE 9.1

Blood Pressure Management

Treatment	Measurement	Recommendations/Comments
Post-thrombolysis	<180/110 mmHg × 24 hours	AHA/ASA guidelines
Post-thrombectomy	<160 mmHg × 24 hours	BP goal is neurosurgeon dependent post operatively
No thrombolysis/No thrombectomy	<220/120 mmHg	AHA/ASA guidelines. Do not attempt to lower BP in acute setting. Areas of ischemia have pressure dependent flow; decrease cerebral perfusion leads to worsening of stroke.

(continued)

TABLE 9.1 (*continued*)

Blood Pressure Management

Hemorrhagic conversion	SBP <140 or <160	Controversial. INTERACT study SBP <140 had hematoma expansion decreased by 22%. AHA/ASA patients with SBP 150–200 mmHg and no contraindications to acute BP management lowering SBP <140 is safe and improves functional outcome.

AHA, American Heart Association; ASA, American Stroke Association; BP, blood pressure; SBP, systolic blood pressure.

FAST FACTS

Ideal blood pressure (BP) is controversial and must take patient's baseline into consideration. Initial BP reduction by 15% is a reasonable goal. A change in mental status with lower systolic blood pressure (SBP) may require pressure-induced hypertension to improve blood flow and decrease neurological consequences of stroke (Powers et al., 2019).

Postthrombolytic Initial Orders

- CT head 24 hours after thrombolytic transfusion; evaluate for hemorrhagic conversion
- Stat CT head if concerns for hemorrhagic conversion: headache, nausea, vomiting, worsening of neurological deficits, and/or altered mental status
- Cardiac monitoring
- Temperature management <99.5°F
- Glycemic control 140 to 180
- Vital signs and neuro checks every 15 minutes × 2 hours, every 30 minutes × 6 hours, then every hour (Powers et al., 2019)

Postthrombolytic Hemorrhagic Conversion Initial Orders

- If thrombolytic transfusing immediately STOP the transfusion
- Stat computed tomography head (CTH) and repeat in 6 hours for stability of hemorrhage
- Assess for increased intracranial pressure (ICP) with particular attention to pupillary size and response and assessment of the Glasgow Coma Scale (GCS)
- Vital signs with neuro checks every 15 minutes to ensure stability
- Stat labs to include prothrombin time (PT), partial thromboplastin time (PTT), platelets, fibrinogen, type, and cross
- SBP goal < 140
- Reversal agents: 10 units of cryoprecipitate IV. Can repeat dose if fibrinogen is <150 mg/dL AND tranexamic acid 1,000 mg IV or aminocaproic acid IV 4 to 5 g and followed by 1 g until bleeding stops
- Consult neurosurgery. If neurosurgery is not available, transfer patient to facility with capability.
- Consider platelet transfusion.

FAST FACTS

Hemorrhagic conversion after ischemic stroke in patients who do not receive thrombolysis is strongly associated with a cardioembolic etiology. Hemorrhagic conversion can occur up to 2 weeks post-thrombolytic.

Angioedema Postthrombolytic Administration

- H-1 blocker diphenhydramine 50 mg intravenous pyelogram (IVP) and H2-blocker ranitidine 50 mg IV or famotidine 20 mg is first line treatment
- If increased edema 100 mg methylprednisolone or nebulized epinephrine (0.1%) 3 mL subcutaneous of nebulizer 0.5 mL
- Bradykinin antagonist, icatibant 30 mg subcutaneous in abdominal wall, repeat 6 hours, maximum of 90 mg in 24 hours, may be considered
- C1 esterase inhibitor, fresh frozen plasma (FFP) may be required as targeted therapy for hereditary angioedema
- Potential airway obstruction may need endotracheal intubation

FAST FACTS

Angioedema usually occurs 30 to 120 minutes after the infusion in 1% to 3% of patients.

Brain Edema and Increased Intracranial Pressure

The Monroe–Kellie doctrine states that the sum volume of brain, blood, and cerebrospinal fluid (CSF) is constant (Table 9.2). An increase in one component

TABLE 9.2

Intracranial Volume Measurements

Component	Volume	Measurement
Cranial	~1,500 mL	
Blood	~1,200 mL	
CSF • Ventricular • CSF production	~250 mL ~125 mL ~250 mL	
CBF	~55 mL (100 g/min)	mL (blood) (tissue/min) CBF = CPP/CVR
CPP		~50–150 mmHg CPP = MAP–ICP
ICP		Normal 7–15 mmHg Goal <20 mmHg

CBF, cerebral blood flow; CPP, cerebral perfusion pressure; CSF, cerebrospinal fluid; CVR, cerebrovascular reactivity; ICP, intracranial pressure; MAP, mean arterial pressure.

must cause a proportional decrease in others. A change in intracranial volume that exceeds the compensation mechanism may displace the brain parenchyma resulting in herniation, as the skull is a rigid compartment.

FAST FACTS

Large ischemic strokes lead to cytotoxic edema and later result in vasogenic edema (Table 9.3). Clinically relevant edema develops 24 to 72 hours after stroke onset.

TABLE 9.3

Differences in Cerebral Edema

	Cytotoxic Edema	Vasogenic Edema
Pathophysiology	Blood–brain barrier intact The failure of Na+ to K+ ATP neuronal channels results in intracellular accumulation of water Occurs within minutes of stroke	Blood–brain barrier is compromised, plasma proteins and intravascular water leak out of endothelial cells into extracellular space
CT	Involves both cortical gray and white matter Gray and white matter junction blurred	■ Confined to white matter ■ Gray and white matter distinction more pronounced ■ Fingerlike extensions involving mainly white matter
MRI	■ DWI hyperintense signal ■ ADC hypointense signal ■ Restricted diffusion	■ Hyperintense T2 and flair signals on white matter ■ Hypointense TI ■ No restricted diffusion
Etiology	Stroke	Benign and malignant neoplasms
Treatment	Osmotic therapy (mannitol or 3% saline) *Corticosteroids not recommended for cerebral edema and/or increased ICP complicating stroke because of the risk of potential harm*	Corticosteroids

ADC, apparent diffusion coefficient; ATP, adenosine triphosphate; DWI, diffusion weighted imaging; ICP, intracranial pressure; TI, therapeutic index.

FAST FACTS

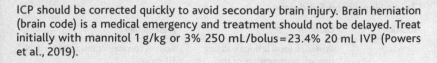

ICP should be corrected quickly to avoid secondary brain injury. Brain herniation (brain code) is a medical emergency and treatment should not be delayed. Treat initially with mannitol 1 g/kg or 3% 250 mL/bolus=23.4% 20 mL IVP (Powers et al., 2019).

Surgical Management

Surgical decompression should be done as soon as any signs of herniation (Table 9.4) develop if there is no response to medical therapy. Cerebellar infarction involves suboccipital decompression. Avoid using ventricular drainage as it may cause upward herniation and does not relieve the direct brainstem compression.

TABLE 9.4

Classic Herniation Syndromes

Location	Cause	Presentation
Subfalcine	Passage of contents of either anterior fossa beneath the falx cerebri	Loss of attention and apathy. Inability to recite days of week months of year.
Diencephalic shift or torsion	Compression and distortion of the thalami and midbrain	Alteration of consciousness, small pupils, lack of posturing with flaccid extremities. Presentation can be mistaken for encephalopathy or coma secondary to toxic/metabolic cause.
Uncal	Volume of middle cranial fossa exceeds its capacity; the temporal lobe uncus herniates into the space occupied by the adjacent ipsilateral CN III, PCA and cerebral peduncle of midbrain.	Ipsilateral CN III palsy localizing feature. As progresses either ipsilateral, contralateral, or bilateral weakness with/without flexor posturing.
Transtentorial/central	Direct upward pressure and displacement of the midline structures, including brainstem, through tentorial notch. The ascending path of CN VI from the rostral pons to the cavernous sinus will have downward traction.	Early clinical feature is asymmetric CN VI palsy. Bilateral upper limb flexion bilateral lower limb extension. As herniation progresses all limbs will have extension reflex then complete absence of motor response.

(continued)

TABLE 9.4 (*continued*)

Classic Herniation Syndromes

Location	Cause	Presentation
Upward	Posterior fossa lesions causing upward compression of the midbrain, thalami and superior cerebellar artery. A critical complication is compression of cerebral aqueduct can lead to obstructive hydrocephalus.	Loss of consciousness, superior CN III palsy
Tonsillar	It can result from any herniation but typically results from posterior fossa lesions. The cerebellar tonsil descends through the foramen magnum with direct compression of the medulla. *Due to the limited space in the posterior fossa of the skull, little edema can cause dangerous tissue compensation with cerebral spinal fluid blockage.*	The classic presentation is Cushing's triad hypertension, reflex bradycardia, and irregular breathing to apnea.

CN, cranial nerves; PCA, patient-controlled analgesia.

FAST FACTS

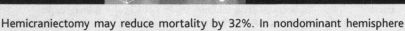

Eighty percent of patients developing signs of brainstem compression will die, usually within hours to days.

Middle cerebral artery territory infarction should be treated with aggressive therapies to reduce morbidity and mortality (Torbey & Selim, 2016).

FAST FACTS

Hemicraniectomy may reduce mortality by 32%. In nondominant hemisphere stroke, hemicraniectomy may reduce hemiplegia, and in dominant hemisphere strokes reduce mild to moderate aphasia if surgery is performed early (prior to herniation).

Hemicraniectomy indications include the following: ≤70 years of age, more strongly indicated in nondominant hemisphere, clinical and CT evidence of acute complete middle artery infarcts, and direct signs of impending or complete severe hemisphere brain edema (Powers et al., 2019).

Airway Management

A patient with impaired level of consciousness, decreased respiratory drive, loss of protective reflexes, and/or dysphagia should be evaluated for endotracheal mechanical ventilation. Independent risk factors for mortality in respiratory failure after ischemic stroke ≥60 years old and Glasgow Coma Scale ≤10 are associated with low probability of survival of 33% two years post stroke.

FAST FACTS

Lung protective principles should be followed. Goals of ventilation should be optimal arterial oxygenation with arterial partial pressure of oxygen (PaO2) ≥70 and normalization of the arterial of carbon dioxide (PaCO2) to between 35 and 40 mmHg as a drop may lead to cerebral vasoconstriction and risk of secondary ischemia.

It is reasonable to consider tracheostomy in acute ischemic stroke patients failing or unable to extubate within seven to 14 days after intubation.

CARDIOVASCULAR EVENTS

Elevated troponins are observed in up to 18% of stroke patients. Some myocardial infarctions (MIs) with non-ST segment elevation events are likely secondary to neurocardiogenic origins. Troponin elevations are less likely in ischemic stroke patients than in hemorrhagic strokes. Avoid cardiac catheterization unless there is imminent need in patients with ST-elevation MI due to the competing interests between the brain and heart in relation with BP management and antithrombotic therapy.

***Caution.* Decompensated congestive heart failure can result when diuretics are held to induce hypertension.**

INFECTIONS

Aspiration-associated pneumonia is present in as many as 22% of stroke patients during their hospitalization. Urinary tract infections are also common and present in 24% during their hospital stay. It is associated with inappropriately prolonged periods of indwelling urinary catheters, as bladder dysfunction is very common in the acute period. A dysphagia screening should be completed before the patient begins eating, drinking, or receiving oral medication to effectively identify patients at risk for aspiration (Powers et al., 2019).

FAST FACTS

According to the American Speech-Language-Hearing Association, screening tests should include capturing a history of dysphagia, diagnosis that affects swallowing (stroke), overt signs of aspiration, complaints of swallowing difficulties, and a pass or fail recommendation.

TEMPERATURE

Hyperthermia (temperature ≥ 38°C) should be identified and treated. Antipyretic medications should be administered to lower temperature in hyperthermic patients with stroke (Powers et al., 2019).

FAST FACTS

To date, studies of hypothermia in ischemic stroke patients showed no benefit in functional outcome and suggest that induction of hypothermia increases risk of infection, including pneumonia.

GLUCOSE

Evidence indicates that persistent in-hospital hyperglycemia during the first 24 hours after ischemic stroke is associated with worse outcomes than normoglycemia. It is reasonable to treat hyperglycemia to achieve blood glucose levels between 140 and 180 mg/dL and to monitor closely to prevent hypoglycemia (Powers et al., 2019).

HEMORRHAGIC STROKE

Hemorrhage stroke is the deadliest form of stroke and occurs in 15% to 30% of strokes. The onset is usually progressive over minutes to hours with symptoms of nausea, vomiting, severe headache, and decreased level of consciousness. The diagnosis and management of a hemorrhagic stroke is a medical emergency. Within the first hours of a patient's arrival to the hospital, 15% to 23% will continue to deteriorate with a high rate of poor long-term outcome, so early aggressive management is imperative (Hinduja & Ahmed, 2019).

Diagnosis and Management

- Baseline severity score; see scales in Chapter 5 (Class I level of evidence [LoE] B; Hemphill et al., 2015)
- Rapid neuroimaging with CT or MRI to distinguish ischemic stroke from hemorrhagic stroke (Class I LoE A; Hemphill et al., 2015)
- Consider CTA and contrast-enhanced CT for risk of hematoma expansion, CT cerebral venogram (CTV), MRI, magnetic resonance angiogram (MRA), and magnetic resonance venogram (MRV) to evaluate structural lesions or vascular malformations (Class IIB LoE B; Hemphill et al., 2015)

Initial Management

Laboratory Tests

- Complete blood count
  - Thrombocytopenia should receive replacement therapy.

- Electrolytes
  - Hyperglycemia is associated with worse prognosis.
  - Monitor for hyponatremia, possible syndrome of inappropriate antidiuretic hormone secretion (SIADH).
    - Avoid rapid correction or overcorrection to reduce risk of osmotic demyelination.
    - Check Na every 4 to 6 hours; do not exceed 8 to 10 mEq/L in 24 hours.
- PT, PTT, international normalized ratio (INR)
  - INR elevated secondary to vitamin K antagonist (VKA); hold VKA and replace with intravenous vitamin K (Class I LoE C; Hemphill et al., 2015).
  - Severe coagulation factor deficiency should receive replacement therapy.
- Troponin: elevation is associated with worse outcome
- Toxicology screen: mainly cocaine and/or adrenergic drugs
- Women of childbearing age obtain pregnancy test

Reversal

- Dabigatran (consider hemodialysis), rivaroxaban, or apixaban, treatment with factor eight inhibitor bypass activity (FEIBA), other prothrombin complex concentrates (PCCs), or rFVIIa may be considered on individual basis. If most recent dose taken < 2 hours, activated charcoal may be considered (Class IIb LoE C; Hemphill et al., 2015).
  - Please see Chapter 10, Critical Care Pharmacology, regarding reversal agents.
- Heparin reversal with protamine (Class IIb LoE C; Hemphill et al., 2015).

FAST FACTS

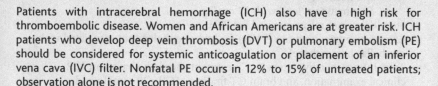

Patients with intracerebral hemorrhage (ICH) also have a high risk for thromboembolic disease. Women and African Americans are at greater risk. ICH patients who develop deep vein thrombosis (DVT) or pulmonary embolism (PE) should be considered for systemic anticoagulation or placement of an inferior vena cava (IVC) filter. Nonfatal PE occurs in 12% to 15% of untreated patients; observation alone is not recommended.

BLOOD PRESSURE MANAGEMENT PRACTICE GUIDELINES (AHA/ASA)

The current evidence reveals early intensive BP lowering is safe and feasible and patients show improved functional outcome.

- SBP between 150 and 200 mmHg on presentation and without contraindication to acute BP treatment, acute lowering of SBP 140 mmHg is safe (Class I LoE A; Hemphill et al., 2015).

In the severely brain injured patient, BP monitoring is essential for prevention and treatment of intracranial hypertension and secondary brain insults. Invasive BP measurement is the gold standard, and an arterial line should be placed in critically ill patients.

NONSURGICAL MANAGEMENT AND PREVENTION OF SECONDARY BRAIN INJURY

- Intubate if stuporous or comatose
- Maintain normothermia (Class IIb LoE C; Hemphill et al., 2015)
- Seizures and antiseizure drugs
  - Patients with a change of mental status should be evaluated for clinical or subclinical seizures with electroencephalogram (EEG).
  - Clinical seizures should be treated with antiseizure medications (ASMs; Class I LoE A; Hemphill et al., 2015).
  - Prophylactic ASM is not routinely recommended (Class III LoE B; Hemphill et al., 2015).
    - New evidence is emerging (PEACH trial) that suggests seizure prophylaxis with levetiracetam may be reasonable.
  - ASM options:
    - First line agents lorazepam 0.1 mg/kg up to 4 mg may repeat 5 to 10 minutes. Preferred initial ASM, longer duration of action 12 to 24 hours midazolam 0.2 mg/kg to max 10 mg, diazepam 0.15 mg/kg up to 10 mg/kg per dose, may repeat in 5 minutes
    - Second line agents loading dose fosphenytoin 20 mg PE/kg IV piggyback (IVPB), levetiracetam 60 mg/kg max dose 4,500 mg, valproate 40 mg/kg IV max dose 3,000 mg, iacosamide 400 mg IV
    - Levetiracetam has a very favorable therapeutic profile; dose 500 mg q12 hours
    - Fosphenytoin load with 17 mg/kg
- Steroids are not recommended for ICH.
- External ventricular drain (EVD) for hydrocephalus (not associated with cerebellar hemorrhage).
- Treat intracranial hypertension. Treatment should be based on ICP, clinical examination, and brain CT findings. ICP < 20 mmHg and CPP > 50 mmHg. Primary goal is to control ICP simultaneously with cerebral perfusion pressure (CPP) while maintaining adequate mean arterial pressure (MAP).
  - General measures (Darsie & Moheet, 2017)
    - Elevate head of bed (HOB) to 30 to 45 degrees. This decreases ICP by enhancing venous outflow, but also reduces mean carotid pressure; there is no change in cerebral blood flow.
    - Keep neck straight; avoid constrictions. Constriction of jugular venous outflow causes increased ICP.
    - Avoid hypoxia PaO2 < 60 Sat < 90%. Hypoxia can cause further brain ischemia.

        - Ventilate to normocarbia ($PaCO_2$ 35 to 40 mmHg). Avoid prophylactic hyperventilation.
        - Noncontrast CTH. Rule out surgical intervention.
    - Specific measures
        - Heavy sedation. Reduces elevated sympathetic tone and hypertension-induced movement.
        - If EVD is in place, drain 3 to 5 mL CSF. Reduces intracranial volume.
        - Mannitol 0.25 to 1 g/kg every 6 hours. Initially increases plasma volume and increases serum tonicity which draws fluid out of the brain and decreases intracranial volume. Avoid this if the patient is hypovolemic (serum osmol >320) and hypotensive. Has diuretic effect.
        - Hypertonic saline 23.4% 20 mL IVP (need central line) or 3% 250 mL bolus. Caution in patients with congestive heart failure or renal insufficiency due to increased fluid and volume loads. Patients' refractory to mannitol will respond to hypertonic saline.
    - Cushing triad with elevated ICP: hypertension, bradycardia, and respiratory irregularity.
- Cardiac monitoring. Continuous monitoring in the ICU. Systemic screening for myocardial ischemia or infarction is recommended. EKG and cardiac enzymes should be checked routinely.

SURGICAL INTERVENTIONS

External ventriculostomy drain (EVD) indications:

- Acute hydrocephalus associated with intraventricular blood clot may cause obstructive hydrocephalus and intraventricular blood alone is a risk for communicating hydrocephalus. Not recommended for cerebellar hemorrhage.
    - Cerebellar hemorrhage with neurological deterioration or brainstem compression and/or obstructive hydrocephalus from clot should be removed surgically as soon as possible.
- ICP management

ADDITIONAL CONDSIDERATIONS

- Early ICH evacuation is not clearly superior to evacuation when the patient deteriorates (Greenburg, 2020).
- In deteriorating patients, ICH evacuation may be considered as a lifesaving measure.
- Patients in coma, large ICH with midline shift, or elevated ICP refractory to medical measurements a decompressive craniotomy with or without ICH evacuation may reduce mortality. See Chapter 8 for surgical management of ICH.

SUBARACHNOID HEMORRHAGE

Subarachnoid hemorrhage (SAH) is the most complex acute condition that we encounter in medicine. The healthcare team must face difficult and important issues associated with not only neurological complications but also many systemic complications, and this requires a multidisciplinary team approach.

FAST FACTS

Aneurysms are the most frequent cause of SAH. In the majority of cases, aneurysms are shown well on angiography, but in 15% to 20% of cases of SAH the angiogram is negative.

What a practitioner should do in these cases is still controversial. Some groups recommend a second or third angiogram since aneurysms can be temporarily thrombosed at the time of bleeding and become visible only on a late angiogram. In some cases, only a slight abnormality of the vessel wall is recognizable.

Clinical Management and Diagnosis

- Aneurysmal subarachnoid hemorrhage (aSAH) is a medical emergency that is frequently misdiagnosed. A high level of suspicion for aSAH should exist in patients with acute onset of severe headache (Class I LoE B; Connolly et al., 2012).
- Noncontract head CT, if nondiagnostic then should be followed by lumbar puncture.
- Head CT angiogram should be considered in the aSAH workup. This study will help guide the decision for type of aneurysm repair. If inconclusive, it should be followed by digital subtraction angiography (DSA; Class IIb LoE C; Connolly et al., 2012).
- MRI is reasonable for the diagnosis of aSAH in patients with nondiagnostic CT; a negative result does not obviate the need for lumbar puncture for CSF analysis (Class IIb LoE C; Connolly et al., 2012).
- DSA is indicated for detection of aneurysm and for planning surgical treatment (Class I LoE B; Connolly et al., 2012).

Initial Management Concerns

Rebleeding is the major concern during the initial stabilization. Risk factors include the following: female gender, high grade SAH, large aneurysm, and SBP >175 mmHg. Factors associated with rebleeding include longer time to aneurysm treatment, worse neurological status on admission, initial loss of consciousness, previous sentinel headache, larger aneurysm size, and possibly SBP >160 mmHg. There is a risk of rebleeding during any period that the aneurysm is untreated. Early treatment of the ruptured aneurysm can reduce the risk of rebleeding. Higher Hunt and Hess grades, larger aneurysm size, and poorly controlled BP >160 mm Hg have been associated with the increased risk of rebleeding. BP goal <140 mm Hg with unsecured aneurysm and <160 mm Hg with secured aneurysm. If BP is labile, nicardipine or clevedipine infusion should be used in conjunction with an arterial line. Consider clevedipine over nicardipine when volume overload is a concern. Labetalol is a second line option. Avoid hypotension as it may exacerbate ischemia (Connolly et al., 2012).

Hydrocephalus developing precipitously may be obstructive due to blockage of CSF flow by blood clot. Ventriculomegaly early after SAH as well as at later stages is often due to communicating hydrocephalus due to toxic effect of blood breakdown products on arachnoid granulations.

- aSAH associated with acute symptomatic hydrocephalus should be managed by CSF diversion (Class I LoE B; Connolly et al., 2012).
- Slow wean of external ventricular device does not appear to be effective in reducing need for ventricular shunting (Class III LoE B; Connolly et al., 2012).

Delayed cerebral ischemia can produce delayed ischemic neurologic deficit usually attributed to vasospasm. Typically, does not occur until several days following SAH.

FAST FACTS

Hyponatremia follows aSAH in 10% to 30% of cases.

The neurological effects of hyponatremia may mimic delayed ischemic neurologic deficit from vasospasm. Hyponatremia patients have three times the incidence of delayed cerebral infarction after SAH than normonatremic patients and have longer hospital stays. Risk factors for hyponatremia after SAH include hx diabetes mellitus (DM), congestive heart failure (CHF), cirrhosis, adrenal insufficiency, or the use of any nonsteroidal antiinflammatory drugs (NSAIDs), acetaminophen, narcotics, or thiazide diuretics. The etiology of hyponatremia may be multifactorial and may differ in specific cases; etiologies include cerebral salt wasting as a result of natriuresis and diuresis. Cerebral salt wasting is the cause of hyponatremia in the majority of aSAH patients. Extracellular fluid volume is low in cerebral salt wasting and is normal or delayed in SIADH. The observed increase in antidiuretic hormone (ADH) after aSAH may be secondary to hypovolemia.

FAST FACTS

The use of fludrocortisone acetate and hypertonic saline solution is reasonable for preventing and correcting hyponatremia.

Seizures

No randomized control trial has been performed to help guide decisions on prophylaxis or treatment of seizures. There is also conflicting evidence on whether onset seizures are predictive of late seizures or post SAH epilepsy. As such there is no consensus amongst practitioners regarding the need for ASMs, the best ASM to use, which patient should receive prophylactic ASMs, or the optimal dose or duration of treatment.

FAST FACTS

Studies have assessed neurological outcomes following short- and long-term phenytoin use with higher doses and longer duration associated with poorer outcomes. When compared to phenytoin, leviteracetam is associated with a higher rate of short-term seizure recurrence but improved long-term outcomes with fewer side effects.

Although use of prophylactic ASMs for aSAH is controversial, a generalized seizure may be devastating in the presence of a tenuous aneurysm. As such, ASMs are given by many practitioners in the acute setting at least until the aneurysm is secured.

Neurogenic Stress Cardiomyopathy

Some patients may develop myocardial hypokinesis following SAH. This may appear comparable with an MI on echocardiogram yet troponin levels are typically lower than would be predicted given the level of myocardial impairment.

FAST FACTS

This condition reverses completely in most cases within five days as normal myocardial cells replace those with defective troponin. However, 10% of patients may progress to an actual MI.

EKG changes in over 50% of cases of SAH include broad or inverted T waves, ST segment elevation or depression, supraventricular tachycardia (SVT), ventricular flutter, ventricular fibrillation, and bradycardia. Possible mechanism elevation of intracranial pressure secondary to SAH is thought to cause sympathetic activation resulting in hypercontraction of cardiac myocytes and subsequent myocardial injury.

Augmenting Cerebral Oxygen Delivery

- Optimize cerebral blood flow.
- Avoid hypotension as it negatively impacts cerebral blood flow. If vasoactive infusion is needed, avoid use in hypovolemic patients. If heart rate is low, use norepinephrine. If heart rate is elevated, use phenylephrine.
- Maintain normal intracranial pressure.
- Avoid induced hypertension. If cerebral autoregulation is intact, increasing CPP has little effect on cerebral blood flow due to increase in cerebral vascular resistance.

- Avoid hypovolemia. Most patients become hypovolemic in the first 24 hours after aSAH. Hypovolemia is associated with vasospasm.
- Elevate oxygen saturation. With patients at risk for delayed cerebral ischemia, the goal is 100%; maintain >92% for all other patients.
- Optimal hemoglobin (Hgb) is controversial.
  - Increasing Hgb increases blood viscosity, which increases cerebral vascular resistance.
  - Current recommendation is Hgb 8 to 10 (Connolly et al., 2012).

MANAGEMENT OF CEREBRAL VASOSPASM

Vasospasm after aSAH is common, occurring most frequently seven to 10 days after aneurysm rupture and resolving spontaneously after 21 days. A vasospasm is the major cause of death and disability in the patients with aSAH.

- Oral nimodipine should be administered to all patients with aSAH (Class I LoE A; Connolly et al., 2012).

FAST FACTS

Nimodipine has been shown to improve neurological outcomes but not cerebral vasospasm.

- Maintain euvolemia and normal circulating blood volume to prevent delayed cerebral ischemia (Class I LoE B; Connolly et al., 2012).
- Prophylactic hypervolemia or balloon angioplasty before the development of angiographic spasm is not recommended.
- Monitor for the development of arterial vasospasm with transcranial doppler.
- CT perfusion or MRI to evaluate for potential brain ischemia (Greenberg, 1999).
- Induction of hypertension is recommended for patients with delayed cerebral ischemia. Avoid if BP elevated at baseline or worsened current cardiac status (Class I LoE B; Connolly et al., 2012).
- Cerebral angioplasty and/or selective intra-arterial vasodilator therapy for symptomatic cerebral vasospasm (Class IIa LoE B; Connolly et al., 2012).

References

Connolly, E. S., Rabinstein, A. A., Carhuapomam, J. R., Derdeyn, C. P., Dion, J., Higashida, R. T., Hoh, B. L., Kirkness, C. J., Naidech, A. M., Ogilvy, C. S., Patel, A. P., Thomposin, B. G., & Vespa, P. (2012). Guidelines for the management of aneurysmal subarachnoid hemorrhage. A guideline for healthcare professionals from the American Heart Association/American Stroke Association. *Stroke*, *43*(6), 1711–1737.

Darsie, M. D., & Moheet, A. M. (2017). *The pocket guide to neurocritical care: A concise reference for the evaluation and management of neurologic emergencies.* Neurocritical Care Society.

Greenburg, M. S. (2020). *Handbook of neurosurgery* (9th ed.). Thieme Medical Publishers, Inc.

Greenberg, J. O. (1999). *Neuroimaging* (2nd ed.). McGraw-Hill.

Hemphill, J. C., Greenberg, S. M., Anderson, G. S., Becker, K., Bendok, B. R., Cushman, M., Fung, G. L., Goldstein, J. N., Macdonald, R. L., Mitchell, P. H., Scott, P. A., Selim, M. H., & Woo, D. (2015). Guidelines for the management of spontaneous intracerebral hemorrhage: A guideline for healthcare professionals from the American Heart Association/American Stroke Association. *Stroke*, *46*(7), 2032–2060.

Hinduja, A., & Ahmed, M. S. (2019). Emergency neurological life support: Acute ischemic stroke. *Neurocritical Care Society*, 1–51.

Powers, H. J., Rabinstein, A. A., Ackerson, T., Adeoye, O. M., Bambakidis, N. C., Becker, K., Biller, J., Brown, M., Demaerschak, B. M., Hoh, B., Jauch, E. C., Kidwell, C. S., Lesie-Mazwi, T. M., Ovbiagele, B., Scott, P. A., Sheth, K. N., Southerland, A. M., Summers, D. V., & Tirschwell, D. L. (2019). Guidelines for the early management of patients with acute ischemic stroke: 2019 update to the 2018 guidelines for the early management of acute ischemic stroke: A guideline for healthcare professionals from the American Heart Association/American Stoke Association. *Stroke*, *50*(12), e314–e418.

Torbey, M. T., & Selim, M. H. (2016). *The stroke book* (2nd ed.). Cambridge University Press.

10

Critical Care Pharmacology

Keaton S. Smetana and Elizabeth J. Legros

Choosing the appropriate pharmacologic agent is imperative in the management of patients with ischemic and hemorrhagic strokes. A basic understanding of the pharmacologic properties, common adverse effects, and dose to use can assist the neurocritical care provider in reaching goals outlined in the care of the patient. This chapter provides basic pharmacologic information and pearls to assist in agent selection. It covers medications commonly used in the setting of stroke: antihypertensives, thrombolytics, bleeding reversal agents, and medications used in refractory vasospasm management in the setting of aneurysmal subarachnoid hemorrhage (ASAH).

ACUTE BLOOD PRESSURE MANAGEMENT

Appropriate blood pressure control may be necessary during the initial presentation of a patient who had an ischemic or hemorrhagic stroke. Blood pressure may need to be reduced to qualify a patient for IV thrombolytic in the ischemic setting or controlled to prevent expansion of a hemorrhagic stroke. A variety of antihypertensive agents are used for acute management in the setting of acute ischemic stroke (AIS) and hemorrhagic stroke/subarachnoid hemorrhage (SAH)/intracerebral hemorrhage (ICH) though the evidence to guide agent choice is currently limited (Laurent, 2017). IV push medications provide more rapid blood pressure reduction without the need of an infusion pump while continuous IV administration is used for sustained blood pressure control. Ideal antihypertensive medications used to lower blood pressure in stroke patients should have rapid onset, simple titration, minimal adverse effects, and a short half-life (Haller et al., 2019).

BETA-BLOCKERS

Beta-blockers work to lower blood pressure by reducing cardiac output and causing vasodilation to varying degrees. This is accomplished by their effects on a combination of beta-1 adrenergic receptors, beta-2 adrenergic receptors, or alpha-1 adrenergic receptors.

Contraindications

- Severe sinus bradycardia
- Heart block greater than first degree
- Sick sinus syndrome
- Decompensated or uncontrolled heart failure
- Cardiogenic shock
- Pulmonary hypertension
- Severe peripheral arterial circulatory disorders
- Coadministration of IV nondihydropyridine calcium channel blockers (e.g., verapamil, diltiazem)
- Known hypersensitivity

Adverse Effects

- Bradycardia
- Dizziness
- Hypotension
- Risk of exacerbating reactive airway disease
- May mask symptoms of hypoglycemia

Esmolol (Brevibloc)

Pertinent Pharmacokinetic Information

- Beta-1 selective adrenergic blocker (cardioselective)
- Steady-state achieved in 5 minutes, if loading dose administered
- Short half-life (9 minutes; Baxter Healthcare Corporation, 2018)

Dose

- Loading dose 250 to 1,000 mcg/kg administered over one minute
- Followed by a continuous infusion starting at 25 to 50 mcg/kg/min (maximum of 300 mcg/kg/min)
- No renal or hepatic dose adjustments are necessary.
  - Metabolism occurs by esterases in red blood cells via hydrolysis of the ester linkage.

FAST FACTS

Studies in pregnancy are limited, and risks versus benefits should be evaluated. Exposure in pregnant women may cause fetal bradycardia.

Labetalol (Normodyne, Trandate)

Pertinent Pharmacokinetic Information

- Blocks alpha-1, beta-1, and beta-2 adrenergic receptors
- Activity of alpha to beta-blockade is approximately 1:3 for oral administration and 1:7 for IV administration

- Maximum antihypertensive effects obtained within 5 to 10 minutes after IV bolus
- Half-life of approximately 5.5 hours (Baxter Healthcare Corporation, 2020)

Dose

- 5 to 20 mg IV push over 1 to 2 minutes
  - In the setting of AIS can be repeated once
  - In the setting of ICH can be repeated every 15 minutes
- Continuous infusion 2 to 8 mg/min
- No dosage adjustments are necessary for renal impairment.
- Use with caution in hepatic impairment as unspecified lower doses may be needed per the manufacturer as it is metabolized into an inactive metabolite.

FAST FACTS

Labetalol is recommended by the American College of Obstetricians and Gynecologists (ACOG, n.d.) for acute, severe hypertension in pregnant women.

Calcium Channel Blockers

Dihydropyridine (DHP) calcium channel blockers (CCBs) can be used for blood pressure management. They block the voltage-dependent L-type calcium channels preventing depolarization of arterial smooth muscle cells, cardiac myocytes, and cardiac nodal tissue. DHPs have higher selectivity for vascular smooth muscle cells than cardiac cells and cause vasodilation of small arteries. In the acute setting, DHPs reduce total peripheral resistance and mean arterial pressure while increasing cardiac output; however, chronic administration will result in cardiac output returning to baseline.

Contraindications

- Severe aortic stenosis

Adverse Effects

- Headache
- Hypotension
- Flushing
- Tachycardia
- Nausea/vomiting
- May exacerbate heart failure

Clevidipine (Cleviprex)

Pertinent Pharmacokinetic Information

- Produces a 4% to 5% systolic blood pressure reduction within 2 to 4 minutes of administration
- Terminal half-life is approximately 15 minutes (Chiesi USA, Inc., 2021)

Dose

- Initiate at 1 to 2 mg/hr IV, double the dose at every 90 seconds
  - As blood pressure approaches goal, increase the dose by less than doubling (e.g., 2–4 mg/hr) every 5 to 10 minutes.
  - Most patients receive a maximum dose of 21 mg/hr, but there is limited experience with short-term dosing as high as 32 mg/hr.
  - Per 24 hour period a maximum volume of 1,000 mL is recommended due to the lipid load (at 0.5 mg/mL a dose <21 mg/hr for 24 hours would exceed this limit).
- No renal or hepatic dose adjustments are necessary.
  - Rapidly metabolized by esterases in the blood and extravascular tissue via hydrolysis of the ester linkage

FAST FACTS

- Additional contraindications to Clevidipine:
  - Allergy to soy or eggs
  - Defective lipid metabolism (i.e., hyperlipidemia, lipoid nephrosis, or acute pancreatitis accompanied by hyperlipidemia)
- Contains 0.2 g of lipid/mL (2.0 kcal/mL)
  - Lipid intake restrictions may be necessary for patients with significant lipid metabolism disorders.
  - Increased triglycerides have been reported.
  - Nutrition:
    - Lipid content should be factored into total parenteral nutrition (TPN) calculations.
    - TPN and enteral nutrition calories administered may need to be adjusted.
  - If patient is also receiving propofol (0.1 g of lipid/mL), recognize the additional lipid content (Fresenius Kabi, 2020).
- Discard unused portion 12 hours after vial puncture.
- Monitor for rebound hypertension for a minimum of 8 hours if infused for an extended period of time and not transitioned to another antihypertensive.
- Studies in pregnancy are limited, and risks versus benefits should be evaluated.

Nicardipine (Cardene)

Pertinent Pharmacokinetic Information

- Plasma concentrations increase rapidly in the first 2 hours of infusion.
  - Steady state is achieved after 24 to 48 hours.
- There is approximately a 50% decrease in concentration once the infusion is stopped for 2 hours (America Regent, Inc., 2020).

Dose

- Initiate IV infusion at 5 mg/hr
- May increase infusion rate by 2.5 mg/hr every 5 to 15 minutes

- Maximum infusion rate of 15 mg/hr
- Titrate slowly in patients with heart failure due to possible negative inotropic effects, impaired hepatic function as drug is metabolized by the liver, or impaired renal function due to slower drug clearance.

FAST FACTS

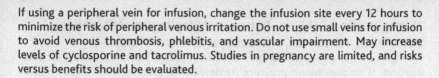

If using a peripheral vein for infusion, change the infusion site every 12 hours to minimize the risk of peripheral venous irritation. Do not use small veins for infusion to avoid venous thrombosis, phlebitis, and vascular impairment. May increase levels of cyclosporine and tacrolimus. Studies in pregnancy are limited, and risks versus benefits should be evaluated.

VASODILATORS

Hydralazine (Apresoline)

Hydralazine causes direct vasodilation of arterioles with minimal effect on venous vasodilation. This results in a reduction of total peripheral resistance (Hikma Pharmaceuticals USA, Inc., 2020).

Contraindications

- Coronary artery disease
- Mitral valvular rheumatic heart disease
- Known hypersensitivity

Adverse Effects

- Tachycardia
- Hypotension
- Edema
- Angina pectoris
- Rash
- Headache
- Nausea, vomiting, diarrhea

Pertinent Pharmacokinetic Information

- Maximum blood pressure reduction occurs in 10 to 80 minutes.
- Half-life of approximately 3 hours; however, blood pressure effects may last 10 to 12 hours.

Dose

- 5 to 20 mg IV push every 30 minutes
- Lower doses may be required in renal impairment.
- No hepatic dose adjustments are required.

FAST FACTS

Hydralazine may be less ideal in AIS compared to other agents because it can increase cerebral ischemia and may cause unpredictable and prolonged drops in blood pressure. However, in the setting of low heart rate (<90 beats/min), it may be an acceptable alternative to labetalol. Hydralazine is recommended by the ACOG for acute, severe hypertension in pregnant women.

Nitroglycerin (GoNitro, Nitrocot, Nitrolingual, NitroMist, Nitroquick, Nitrostat, Nitrotab, and Nitro-Time)

Nitroglycerin is a potent venous vasodilator. High doses can cause arterial dilation. It reduces blood pressure by decreasing preload and cardiac output (Baxter Healthcare Corporation, 2016).

Contraindications

- Increased intracranial pressure (ICP)
- Concomitant use of phosphodiesterase inhibitors (e.g., sildenafil, tadalafil, and vardenafil)
- Concomitant riociguat use
- Known hypersensitivity

Adverse Effects

- Headache
- Hypotension
- Reflex tachycardia
- Tachyphylaxis
- Methemoglobinemia (rare)

Pertinent Pharmacokinetic Information

- Rapid onset (2–5 minutes)
- Short half-life (3 minutes)

Dose

- Initiate a continuous infusion at 5 mcg/min and titrate every 3 to 5 minutes to a maximum rate of 200 mcg/min.
- No renal or hepatic dose adjustments are necessary.

FAST FACTS

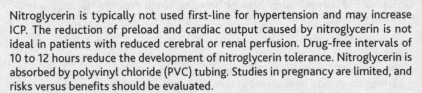

Nitroglycerin is typically not used first-line for hypertension and may increase ICP. The reduction of preload and cardiac output caused by nitroglycerin is not ideal in patients with reduced cerebral or renal perfusion. Drug-free intervals of 10 to 12 hours reduce the development of nitroglycerin tolerance. Nitroglycerin is absorbed by polyvinyl chloride (PVC) tubing. Studies in pregnancy are limited, and risks versus benefits should be evaluated.

Sodium Nitroprusside (Nipride, Nitropress, and Sodium Nitroprusside)

Sodium nitroprusside is a potent arterial and venous vasodilator. It decreases both afterload and preload.

Contraindications

- Compensatory hypertension, where the primary hemodynamic lesion is aortic coarctation or arteriovenous shunting
- Do not use to produce hypotension during surgery in known inadequate cerebral circulation, or in moribund patients (American Society of Anesthesiologists [ASA] Class 5E) requiring emergency surgery (Xiromed, LLC, 2021).
- Congenital (Leber's) optic atrophy or tobacco amblyopia
- Acute congestive heart failure associated with reduced systemic vascular resistance (i.e., septic shock)
- Concomitant use of phosphodiesterase inhibitors (e.g., sildenafil, tadalafil, and vardenafil)
- Concomitant riociguat use
- Known hypersensitivity

Adverse Effects

- Flushing
- Increased intracranial pressure
- Methemoglobinemia (rare)
- Thiocyanate toxicity (rare)

Pertinent Pharmacokinetic Information

- Rapid onset within a few seconds
- Short half-life (3 minutes)

Dose

- Per the package prescribing information:
  - Initiate infusion at 0.3 mcg/kg/min and titrate every 5 minutes to effect
  - Maximum recommended infusion rate of 10 mcg/kg/min
    - Terminate infusion immediately if blood pressure not controlled after 10 minutes at maximum infusion rate.
- Use with caution in renal impairment as thiocyanate may accumulate.
  - Nitroprusside combines with hemoglobin to produce cyanide and cyanmethemoglobin. Cyanide is then converted to thiocyanate which is eliminated in the urine.
- Use with caution in hepatic impairment.

FAST FACTS

- Boxed warnings:
  - Not for direct injection; must be diluted
  - Precipitous decreases in blood pressure; requires continuous blood pressure monitoring
  - Risk of cyanide toxicity
    - Increased risk at rates above 2 mcg/kg/min
    - At higher infusion rates, thiosulfate may be coadministered to mitigate cyanide toxicity.
- Sodium nitroprusside decreases cerebral blood flow while increasing intracranial pressure.
  - Not an ideal agent for hypertension unless all other treatment options have failed or are unavailable due to risks of rebound hypertension, cyanide toxicity, and potential to raise intracranial pressure
- Protect product from light.
- Studies in pregnancy are limited, and risks versus benefits should be evaluated.

Other Antihypertensive Agents

Clonidine (Catapres, Catapres-TTS, Duraclon, Jenloga, and Kapvay)

Clonidine is an alpha-2 adrenergic agonist. It stimulates alpha-2 adrenoceptors in the brainstem to reduce sympathetic outflow which decreases norepinephrine plasma concentrations providing a reduction in blood pressure. Clonidine decreases both cardiac output and total peripheral resistance (Actavis Pharma, Inc., 2015).

Contraindications

- Known hypersensitivity

Adverse Effects

- Sedation
- Fatigue
- Headache
- Rash
- Dry mouth
- Decreased libido
- Vivid dreams and sleep disturbance
- Symptomatic bradycardia
- Atrioventricular blocks
- Withdrawal

Pertinent Pharmacokinetic Information

- Peak levels of clonidine in 1 to 3 hours
- Half-life of 12 to 16 hours

Dose

- Oral initial dose of 0.1 mg twice daily (max dose 2.4 mg/d)
- Sublingual administration described off-label:
  - Initial dose 0.1 to 0.2 mg, followed by 0.5 to 0.1 mg every hour to a max dose of 0.7 mg
- Lower doses may be required in renal impairment.
- No dose adjustments are recommended for hepatic impairment.

FAST FACTS

Transdermal patches have a delayed time to therapeutic onset and should not be used in the acute setting of blood pressure management. Studies in pregnancy are limited, and risks versus benefits should be evaluated.

Enalaprilat (Enalaprilat, Epaned, Vasotec, and Vasotec)

Enalaprilat is an angiotensin converting enzyme inhibitor (ACEI) that prevents the conversion of angiotensin I to angiotensin II. This decrease in angiotensin II, a vasoconstrictor, results in vasodilation of small resistance arteries. ACEIs reduce total peripheral resistance while maintaining cardiac output (West-Ward Pharmaceutical Corp., 2010).

Contraindications

- History of angioedema due to ACEIs
- Hereditary or idiopathic angioedema
- Pregnancy
- Known hypersensitivity

Adverse Effects

- Cough
- Angioedema (rare)
- Hypotension
- Hyperkalemia
- Renal failure
- Hepatic failure

Pertinent Pharmacokinetic Information

- Enalaprilat is the active metabolite of enalapril.
- Onset of action in about 15 minutes; maximum effect in 1 to 4 hours
- Half-life of approximately 11 hours

Dose

- Administer 1.25 mg IV push over 5 minutes every 6 hours.
  - Doses as high as 5 mg every 6 hours were tolerated.
  - If patients are receiving diuretics, recommend initiation at 0.625 mg.
- If creatinine clearance is ≤30 mL/min, initiate dose at 0.625 mg.
- No dose adjustments are required for hepatic impairment.

FAST FACTS

Use caution in the setting of thrombolytic administration (alteplase and tenecteplase) as enalaprilat may increase the risk of orolingual angioedema. Use in pregnancy is contraindicated.

Phentolamine (Phentolamine Mesylate, Oraverse)

Phentolamine is an alpha-adrenergic blocker. It has positive inotropic and chronotropic effects on cardiac muscle and vasodilator effects on vascular smooth muscle (Precision Dose, Inc., 2017).

Contraindications

- Myocardial infarction or history of myocardial infarction
- Coronary insufficiency
- Angina or other signs of coronary artery disease
- Known hypersensitivity

Adverse Effects

- Tachycardia
- Hypotension
- Cardiac arrhythmias
- Dizziness
- Flushing
- Nausea, vomiting, and diarrhea

Pertinent Pharmacokinetic Information

- Half-life of 19 minutes

Dose

- IV bolus of 5 to 10 mg, additional bolus every 10 minutes to achieve blood pressure target
- No renal or hepatic dose adjustments are necessary.

FAST FACTS

Phentolamine is generally used in settings of catecholamine excess (i.e., pheochromocytoma). Myocardial infarction, cerebrovascular spasm, and cerebrovascular occlusion have been reported after administration of phentolamine, usually due to severe hypotension. Studies in pregnancy are limited, and risks versus benefits should be evaluated.

THROMBOLYTIC THERAPY

Thrombolytic medications result in fibrinolysis of a thrombus by binding to fibrin and converting plasminogen to plasmin. Alteplase is the only approved thrombolytic for reperfusion in AIS. However, tenecteplase has characteristics that may provide advantages over alteplase with less complex administration, a longer half-life, and a higher affinity for fibrin binding (Powers et al., 2019).

Contraindications

- Active internal bleeding
  - Including current intracranial hemorrhage or subarachnoid hemorrhage
- Recent (within 3 months) intracranial or intraspinal surgery
- Recent (within 3 months) serious head trauma
- Intracranial conditions that may increase the risk of bleeding (e.g., aneurysm, arteriovenous malformation, and neoplasm)
- Bleeding diathesis
- Current severe uncontrolled hypertension

Adverse Effects

- Bleeding (sometimes fatal)
- Thromboembolism
- Known hypersensitivity
  - Includes angioedema to thrombolytic (concomitant use of ACEIs may increase the risk)

Alteplase (TPA, Actilyse, Activase, and Cathflo)

Pertinent Pharmacokinetic Information

- A recombinant tissue plasminogen activator (tPA; Genentech, Inc., 2022)
- Decreases circulating fibrinogen by 16% to 36%
- Half-life <5 minutes

Dose

- 0.9 mg/kg (not to exceed 90 mg total dose) IV as a 60 minute infusion with 10% of the total dose administered as an initial bolus over 1 minute
- No renal or hepatic dose adjustments are necessary.

FAST FACTS

Concomitant use of anticoagulants and medications that inhibit platelet function increase the risk of bleeding. May be used within 8 hours of reconstitution when stored at 2°C to 30°C (36°F–86°F). Studies in pregnancy are limited, and risks versus benefits should be evaluated.

Tenecteplase (TNKase)

Pertinent Pharmacokinetic Information

- A modified recombinant tissue plasminogen activator
- Decreases circulating fibrinogen by 4% to 15% (Genentech, Inc., 2018)
- Half-life of 20 to 24 minutes
  - Terminal half-life 90 to 130 minutes

Dose

- IV bolus of 0.25 mg/kg; maximum 25 mg
- No renal or hepatic dose adjustments are necessary.

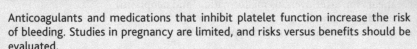

FAST FACTS

Anticoagulants and medications that inhibit platelet function increase the risk of bleeding. Studies in pregnancy are limited, and risks versus benefits should be evaluated.

BLEEDING REVERSAL AGENTS

Oral anticoagulant-related bleeding is a common adverse drug event encountered in the emergency department. While the rate of warfarin-related bleeds has decreased, there has also been an increase in the number of bleeds associated with direct oral anticoagulants with prescribing changes over the last decade. Therefore, it is important to understand the various agents available to reverse the oral anticoagulants on the market. In the setting of warfarin, associated bleeding international normalized ratio (INR) can be used as a guide to dosing. In the setting of direct oral anticoagulants (apixaban, rivaroxaban, dabigatran, etc.), guidelines recommend administering a reversal agent if within 3 to 5 terminal half-lives of the medication. In general, reversal should be considered if the last dose is taken within 48 hours for direct oral anticoagulants. Renal function may impact clearance of these medications and should especially be taken into consideration with dabigatran as it is largely renally eliminated. Additional considerations should be given as to the dose to be administered for direct oral anticoagulants based on the location and size of the bleed and reason for anticoagulation (atrial fibrillation vs. segmental pulmonary embolism; Broderick et al., 2007).

Andexanet Alfa (Coagulation Factor Xa [Recombinant], Inactivated-Zhzo) (Annexa, Andexxa)

Andexanet alfa was approved in 2018 by the U.S. Food and Drug Administration (FDA) for patients treated with rivaroxaban or apixaban, when reversal of anticoagulation is needed due to life-threatening or uncontrolled bleeding (Alexion Pharmaceuticals, Inc., 2022).

Mode of Action and Pertinent Pharmacokinetic Information

- Binds and sequesters the FXaI (rivaroxaban or apixaban)
- Binds and inhibits the activity of tissue factor pathway inhibitor increasing tissue factor-initiated thrombin generation
- Rapid onset of action (minutes)
- Half-life 4.7 hours

Dose

- No renal or hepatic dosing adjustments are necessary.

Factor Xa Inhibitor	Last Dose	Administered <8 hours or at an unknown time	Administered ≥8 hours
Apixaban (Eliquis)	≤5 mg	Low Dose	Low Dose
	>5 mg/unknown	High Dose	
Rivaroxaban (Xarelto)	≤10 mg	Low Dose	
	>10 mg/unknown	High Dose	

Dose	Initial IV Bolus	Following IV Infusion[a]
Low Dose	400 mg Administered over 14 minutes	4 mg/min for up to 120 minutes (480 mg total)
High Dose	800 mg Administered over 27 minutes	8 mg/min for up to 120 minutes (960 mg total)

[a]Infusion should be initiated within 2 minutes of the bolus dose.

Contraindications

- None listed in the package insert

Adverse Reactions

- Thromboembolic or ischemic events
- Infusion related reactions (flushing, feeling hot, cough, dysgeusia, and dyspnea)

FAST FACTS

- A 0.2 or 0.22 micron inline polyethersulfone or equivalent low protein-binding filter should be used with administration.
- Reconstituted andexanet alfa is stable at room temperature for up to 8 hours.
- Dissolution time for each vial is approximately 3 to 5 minutes. The low-dose regimen uses five 200 mg vials and the high-dose regimen uses nine 200 mg vials.

Idarucizumab (Praxbind)

Idarucizumab was approved in 2015 by the U.S. FDA for patients treated with dabigatran (Pradaxa), when reversal of anticoagulation is needed for a) emergency surgery/urgent procedures or b) life-threatening or uncontrolled bleeding (Boehringer Ingelheim Pharmaceuticals, 2015).

Mode of Action and Pertinent Pharmacokinetic Information

- Humanized monoclonal antibody fragment that binds to dabigatran and its metabolites with higher affinity than that of dabigatran to endogenous thrombin. Dabigatran has a half-life of 12 to 17 hours in normal renal function but is prolonged in the setting of renal dysfunction.
- Rapid onset of action
- Half-life elimination: 47 minutes (initial), 10 hours (terminal)
- Renally excreted

Dose

- 5 g, provided as two separate vials that each contain 2.5 g/50 mL
- Administer each vial over 5 to 10 minutes sequentially with the second vial administered no later than 15 minutes after the first vial has finished infusing.
- While data is limited, the package insert states that in patients with elevated coagulation parameters and reappearance of clinically relevant bleeding or requiring a second emergency surgery/urgent procedure, an additional 5 g dose may be considered.

Contraindications

- None listed in the package insert

Adverse Reactions

- Thromboembolic risk
- Headache
- Hypokalemia
- Delirium
- Constipation
- Pyrexia
- Hypersensitivity reaction

FAST FACTS

Reevaluation of coagulation parameters (e.g., activated partial thromboplastin time [aPTT]) may be warranted every 6 hours for at least the first 24 hours after administration to assess the need for additional dosing. Vials are already reconstituted, and no further dilution is warranted. Flush preexisting IV line with .9% sodium chloride prior to infusing idarucizumab.

Four-Factor Prothrombin Complex Concentrate (Beriplex, Confidex, Kcentra, Octaplex, and Profilnine)

Four-factor prothrombin complex concentrate (4F-PCC) was approved for the urgent reversal of acquired coagulation factor deficiency induced by vitamin K antagonist (e.g., warfarin) therapy in adult patients with acute major bleeding.

Mode of Action and Pertinent Pharmacokinetic Information

- Contains the vitamin K-dependent coagulation factors II, VII, IX, and X in addition to antithrombotic proteins C and S. The administration of 4F-PCC rapidly increases the plasma levels of the vitamin K-dependent coagulation factors that are depleted when on a vitamin K antagonist.
- Rapid onset of action. In one study with a median baseline INR of 3.9, a reduction to an INR of 1.2 was observed at 30 minutes.
- Half-life is dependent upon each factor: factor II—60 hours, factor X—31 hours, factor IX—17 hours, and factor VII—4 hours.

Dose

- Based on factor IX component. While vials have labeled amount (e.g., 500 units), each vial may differ slightly in the amount of factor IX.
- Warfarin reversal

Pretreatment INR	2 to <4	4 to 6	<6
Dose of 4F-PCC (Kcentra)	25 units/kg	35 units/kg	50 units/kg
Maximum dose	2,500 units	3,500 units	5,000 units

  - In the setting of ICH, guidelines recommend INR <1.4.
    - If INR is between 1.4 and 1.9, guideline recommendation is dose of 25 units/kg (although 10 units/kg is reasonable)
- Factor Xa inhibitor reversal—apixaban (Eliquis) and rivaroxaban (Xarelto)
  - 50 units/kg (max 5,000 units) in the setting of intracranial hemorrhage if within 3 to 5 terminal half-lives of drug exposure or in the context of liver failure
    - Rivaroxaban half-life: 5 hours
    - Apixaban half-life: 12 hours

Contraindications

- Known anaphylactic or severe systemic reactions to Kcentra or any components of Kcentra which includes heparin; factors VII, IX, X, II; proteins C and S; antithrombin III; and human albumin (CSL Behring, 2020)
- Patients with disseminated intravascular coagulation
- Patients with known heparin-induced thrombocytopenia (HIT)
  - Kcentra 500 unit vials contain 8 to 40 units of heparin. 5,000 units of Kcentra can contain 80 to 400 units of heparin.

Adverse Reactions

- Arterial and venous thromboembolic complications have been reported (stroke, pulmonary embolism, and deep vein thrombosis).
- Headache
- Nausea/vomiting
- Arthralgia
- Hypotension

FAST FACTS

Given the variability in the factor IX component in each vial, the actual dose administered may differ slightly from the dose required. Each 500-unit vial ranges from 400 to 620 factor IX units. For example, if the dose required is 1,500 units but the three 500-unit vials consist of 493 units, 506 units, and 512 units, it would be appropriate to give the three vials together for a dose of 1,511 units. Kcentra contains heparin, and in the package insert a history of HIT is listed as a contraindication. It's important to discuss the risk versus benefit of administering Kcentra in those with HIT. Administration rate is 210 units/min.

Tranexamic Acid (Cyklokapron, Lysteda)

Tranexamic acid (TXA) is an antifibrinolytic indicated in patients with hemophilia to reduce or prevent hemorrhage and reduce the need for replacement therapy during and following tooth extraction. It is listed as an alternative agent to cryoprecipitate in the setting of thrombolytic-associated (alteplase or tPA) intracranial hemorrhage (Execla Pharma Sciences, 2019).

Mode of Action and Pertinent Pharmacokinetic Information

- Synthetic lysine amino acid derivative, which diminishes the dissolution of hemostatic fibrin by plasmin. In the presence of TXA, the lysine receptor binding sites of plasmin for fibrin are occupied, preventing binding to fibrin monomers, stabilizing the fibrin matrix structure.

Dose

- 10 to 15 mg/kg IV over 20 minutes (guideline recommendation)

Contraindications

- Active intravascular clotting
- Hypersensitivity to TXA or any of the ingredients

Adverse Reactions

- Thromboembolic risk
- Seizures (most commonly observed in cardiovascular surgery)
- Gastrointestinal disturbances

FAST FACTS

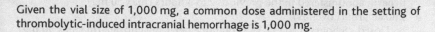

Given the vial size of 1,000 mg, a common dose administered in the setting of thrombolytic-induced intracranial hemorrhage is 1,000 mg.

Vitamin K (Phytonadione)

Mode of Action and Pertinent Pharmacokinetic Information

- Normalizes the INR from vitamin K antagonists (warfarin) by providing the substrate needed to synthesize vitamin K dependent coagulation factors (II, VII, IX, and X; Teligent Pharma, Inc., 2018)

Dose

- 10 mg IV administered over 10 to 20 minutes (max rate of infusion 1 mg/min)

Contraindications

- Hypersensitivity to any component of this medication per the package insert

Adverse Reactions

- Anaphylactoid reactions (incidence is 3 per 10,000 doses)
- Diaphoresis
- Dizziness
- Dysgeusia
- Dyspnea
- Flushing
- Hypotension
- Tachycardia

FAST FACTS

IV administration is the preferred route of administration. IV provides expedited reversal over oral and avoids the reduced bioavailability of subcutaneous administration. Vitamin K should not be used as the sole agent for reversal in the setting of life-threatening bleeds given the time it takes to normalize INR (up to 24 hours).

Protamine Sulfate (Protamine)

Mode of Action and Pertinent Pharmacokinetic Information

- Protamine binds to heparin and heparinoid products to form a stable salt resulting in the loss of anticoagulant activity.
- Neutralization occurs within 5 minutes after IV administration (Fresenius Kabi Ltd, 2016).

Dose

- Unfractionated heparin (UFH): 1 mg IV of protamine for every 100 units of heparin administered in the previous 2 to 3 hours (max 50 mg)
- Enoxaparin (Lovenox):
  - Dosed <8 hours: 1 mg IV of protamine per 1 mg enoxaparin (max 50 mg)
  - Dosed 8 to 12 hours: 0.5 mg IV of protamine per 1 mg enoxaparin (max 50 mg)
    - Minimal utility in administering if dose received beyond 12 hours unless in the setting of acute kidney injury

Contraindications

- Contraindicated in patients who have shown previous intolerance to the drug

Adverse Reactions

- Bleeding or hyperheparinemia has been reported in animal studies and after cardiopulmonary bypass despite neutralization of heparin. Given the anticoagulant effects of protamine, the package insert recommends not administering more than 100 mg over a short period of time.
- Too-rapid of administration can cause severe hypotension and anaphylactoid-like reactions.
- Infertile or vasectomized men may develop antiprotamine antibodies which can result in untoward reactions from protamine.
- Patients with a fish allergy may develop hypersensitivity reactions to protamine due to it being derived from the sperm of salmon. However, no relationship has been established between protamine and fish resulting in an allergic reaction.

FAST FACTS

- Administration rates:
  - Dose ≤15 mg: can be given undiluted by IV push over 3 minutes
  - Dose >15 mg: dilute in 50 mL of 0.9% sodium chloride as an IV piggyback at a maximum rate of 5 mg/min
- Monitor aPTT after administration to ensure reversal has been achieved.

VASOSPASM MANAGEMENT IN ANEURYSMAL SUBARACHNOID HEMORRHAGE

Medications below have been described in the setting of refractory vasospasm in the setting of ASAH. Routes of administration include intravenous, intra-arterial (IA), and intraventricular (IVT) and are described within each medication.

Magnesium Sulfate (MGSO4)

Mode of Action and Pertinent Pharmacokinetic Information

- Thought to provide neuroprotection through inhibiting excitatory pathways (N-methyl-D-aspartate [NMDA] and calcium channels) and may reduce the incidence of vasospasm and subsequent delayed ischemic neurologic deficit (Smetana et al., 2020)

Dose

- Bolus: 4 to 6 g IV
- Continuous infusion: initiate at 0.5 g/hr, titrated to a goal serum magnesium level of 2 to 4 mg/dL

Adverse Reactions

- Flushing
- Hypotension
- Hypermagnesemia
- Hypocalcemia

FAST FACTS

Given lack of evidence in preventing vasospasm, magnesium is usually not used prophylactically.

Milrinone (Primacor)

Mode of Action and Pertinent Pharmacokinetic Information

- Selective inhibitor of cyclic adenosine monophosphate (cAMP) phosphodiesterase (PDE) isozyme III resulting in vasodilation. Additionally, it has inotropic activity due to increasing intracellular ionized calcium in cardiac muscle (Smetana et al., 2020).
- Potentially mitigates vasospasm through the relaxation of cerebral vasculature and increases cerebral perfusion pressure through its inotropic effects.

Dose

- Intravenous:
  - Bolus: 0.1 to 0.2 mg/kg
  - Continuous infusion: 0.5 to 1.5 mcg/kg/min
- IA:
  - 5 to 15 mg infused over 5 to 30 minutes

Adverse Effects
- Hypotension
- Tachycardia
- Ventricular arrhythmias

FAST FACTS

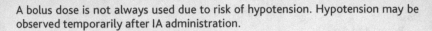

A bolus dose is not always used due to risk of hypotension. Hypotension may be observed temporarily after IA administration.

Nicardipine (Cardene)

Mode of Action and Pertinent Pharmacokinetic Information
- Calcium channel blocker that inhibits the transmembrane influx of calcium ions into cardiac and smooth muscle without changing serum calcium concentrations (Smetana et al., 2020)
- Half-life: 45 minutes

Dose
- IA
  - 2 to 25 mg infused at a rate of 1 mL/min
- Intraventricular
  - 4 mg instilled every 8 to 12 hours

Adverse Effects
- Hypotension
- ICP elevation

FAST FACTS

During IVT administration it is important to withdraw an equal amount of volume to that which will be delivered into the ventricular system. Goal clamp time of the external ventricular drain (EVD) is 30 minutes to 1 hour, but should be allowed to drain earlier if a rise in ICP is observed. Hypotension may be observed temporarily after IA administration.

Verapamil (Isoptin, Calan, Covera, Verap, Verapamil, and Verelan)

Mode of Action and Pertinent Pharmacokinetic Information
- Calcium channel blocker that inhibits the transmembrane influx of calcium ions across cell membranes of the arterial smooth muscle as well as myocardial cells (Smetana et al., 2020)

Dose

- 2.5 to 10 mg infused intra-arterially over 5 to 10 minutes

Common Adverse Effects

- Hypotension

FAST FACTS

Hypotension may be observed temporarily after IA administration.

OSMOTHERAPY AGENTS

Osmotherapy agents are a cornerstone of therapy in the management of elevations in ICP. The general mechanisms which drive ICP reduction after administration of them are that they induce a rapid increase in plasma volume, reduced viscosity and increased deformability of blood cells, and cerebral vasoconstriction. Ultimately, this results in improved cerebral blood flow through the microvasculature and a reduction in ICP (Cook et al., 2020).

Hypertonic Sodium Solutions

Hypertonic sodium solutions are comprised of 3% and 23.4% sodium chloride (saline) and 8.4% sodium bicarbonate.

Dose and Administration Rate

- 3% sodium chloride
  - Emergent ICP reduction:
    - Dose: 250 mL (4–5 mL/kg in pediatrics)
    - Administration: 999 mL/hr on a pump via peripheral IV (PIV) or central access
  - Inducing mild to moderate hypernatremia:
    - Dose: variable
    - Administration: max 80 mL/hr via PIV due to risk of phlebitis and extravasation. If central access is not available, the PIV should be above the wrist in the largest vessel with the smallest bore IV.
- 23.4% sodium chloride
  - Dose: 30 mL
  - Administration: 5 to 10 minutes via central access
    - More data is needed to support the safety of PIV and intraosseous (IO) administration, but a study found it to be safe in their study cohort (Faiver et al., 2021).
- 8.4% sodium bicarbonate
  - Dose: 1 mL/kg administered via PIV or central access
    - Two 50 mL prefilled Abboject syringes
    - Not commonly used as an initial agent for ICP reduction but can be obtained from a crash cart if in an area where other hyperosmolar agents may be delayed in getting to bedside

Adverse Reactions

- Hyperchloremia
- Hypernatremia
- Hypervolemia
- Phlebitis
- Extravasation

FAST FACTS

- Once serum sodium is >165 mEq, the impact on ICP reduction may be diminished with further dosing of hypertonic sodium solutions. An alternative agent such as mannitol can be considered.
- 3% sodium chloride can be administered via PIV for emergent ICP management.
- In patients who become hyperchloremic (>110 mEq), a mixed solution of sodium chloride and sodium acetate can be compounded to reduce the chloride burden.

20% Mannitol (Osmitrol)

Dose

- Emergent ICP reduction: 0.5 to 2.5 g/kg
  - Administered at 999 mL/hr via central access or PIV; must use a 0.22 micron inline filter due to risk of crystallization of the product

Adverse Reactions

- Renal failure
- Hypernatremia
- Electrolyte abnormalities
- Rebound ICP issues

FAST FACTS

20% mannitol contains 20 g of mannitol per 100 mL. A 250 mL bag will have 50 g of mannitol, so two bags (100 g) is the common starting dose in adult patients. Doses less than 0.5 g/kg appear to have a reduced efficacy and duration of action. Given the ability of mannitol to cause rebound ICP issues, it is not administered as a continuous infusion. Mannitol can induce renal injury, and osmolar gap (OG) is used as a surrogate maker of risk. An OG <20 mOsm/kg appears to be a safe cutoff; however, studies have shown a much higher OG to not induce renal failure. In an emergent situation where ICP reduction is needed, the risk and benefit of the therapy should be discussed. If crystals are present in the bag, do not throw them away. These can go back into the solution by gently warming the bag, but it does take time for this to occur. In an emergent situation, it is best to obtain another bag without crystals to not delay administration.

References

Actavis Pharma, Inc. (2015). *Clonidine hydrochloride.* https://dailymed.nlm.nih.gov/dailymed/fda/fdaDrugXsl.cfm?setid=a842ab83-3531-44dd-a8a8-64dd89e87026&type=display

Alexion Pharmaceuticals, Inc. (2022). *Andexanet alfa (Andexxa®).* https://www.andexxa.com/content/dam/open-digital/andexxa-hcp/en/pdf/pi-andexxa-HCP.pdf

American College of Obstetricians and Gynecologists. (n.d.). *Severe hypertension.* https://www.acog.org/community/districts-and-sections/district-ii/programs-and-resources/safe-motherhood-initiative/severe-hypertension

America Regent, Inc. (2020). *Nicardipine hydrochloride injection.* https://americanregent.com/media/3216/nicardipine-insert-rq1087-b-rev-5-2020.pdf

Baxter Healthcare Corporation. (2016). *Nitroglycerin in dextrose.* https://dailymed.nlm.nih.gov/dailymed/fda/fdaDrugXsl.cfm?setid=457a026c-ebce-4701-9deb-2d7652759a99&type=display

Baxter Healthcare Corporation. (2018). *Esmolol hydrochloride injection (Brevibloc).* https://baxterpi.com/pi-pdf/Brevibloc_PI.pdf

Baxter Healthcare Corporation. (2020). *Labetalol hydrochloride injection.* https://baxterpi.com/pi-pdf/Labetalol%20Hydrochloride%20Injection%20PI%2007-19-00-2758%20July%202020.pdf

Boehringer Ingelheim Pharmaceuticals. (2015). *Idarucizumab (Praxbind®).* https://www.accessdata.fda.gov/drugsatfda_docs/nda/2015/761025Orig1s000Approv.pdf

Broderick, J., Connolly, S., Feldmann, E., Hanley, D., Kase, C., Krieger, D., Mayberg, M., Morgenstern, L., Ogilvy, C. S., Vespa, P., Zuccarello, M., American Heart Association/American Stroke Association Stroke Council, American Heart Association/American Stroke Association High Blood Pressure Research Council, & Quality of Care and Outcomes in Research Interdisciplinary Working Group. (2007). Guidelines for the management of spontaneous intracerebral hemorrhage in adults: 2007 update: A guideline from the American Heart Association/American Stroke Association stroke council, high blood pressure research council, and the quality of care and outcomes in research interdisciplinary working group. *Circulation, 116*(16), e391–e413. https://doi.org/10.1161/CIRCULATIONAHA.107.183689

Chiesi USA, Inc. (2021). *Clevidipine (Cleviprex).* https://resources.chiesiusa.com/Cleviprex/CLEVIPREX_US_PI.pdf

Cook, A. M., Morgan Jones, G., Hawryluk, G., Mailloux, P., McLaughlin, D., Papangelou, A., Samuel, S., Tokumaru, S., Venkatasubramanian, C., Zacko, C., Zimmermann, L. L., Hirsch, K., & Shutter, L. (2020). Guidelines for the acute treatment of cerebral edema in neurocritical care patients. *Neurocritical Care, 32*(3), 647–666. https://doi.org/10.1007/s12028-020-00959-7

CSL Behring. (2020). *Kcentra.* https://www.accessdata.fda.gov/drugsatfda_docs/label/2018/012223s042lbl.pdf

Execla Pharma Sciences. (2019). *Tranexamic acid.* https://www.accessdata.fda.gov/drugsatfda_docs/label/2019/212020lbl.pdf

Faiver, L., Hensler, D., Rush, S. C., Kashlan, O., Williamson, C. A., & Rajajee, V. (2021). Safety and efficacy of 23.4% sodium chloride administered via peripheral venous access for the treatment of cerebral herniation and intracranial pressure elevation. *Neurocritical Care, 35*(3), 845–852. https://doi.org/10.1007/s12028-021-01248-7

Fresenius Kabi Ltd. (2016). *Protamine sulphate.* https://www.fresenius-kabi.com/en-ca/documents/Protamine_Sulfate-PI-eng-v1.1-Clean.pdf

Fresenius Kabi. (2020). *Propofol (Diprivan).* https://diprivan-us.com/wp-content/uploads/US-PH-Diprivan_FK-AU451575A_Jan_2020_Austria-PI.pdf

Genentech, Inc. (2018). *Tenecteplase (TNKase).* https://dailymed.nlm.nih.gov/dailymed/fda/fdaDrugXsl.cfm?setid=739a3c53-caf6-40d6-a6af-84ce733a948b&type=display

Genentech, Inc. (2022). *Alteplase (Activase)*. https://dailymed.nlm.nih.gov/dailymed/fda/fdaDrugXsl.cfm?setid=c669f77c-fa48-478b-a14b-80b20a0139c2&type=display

Haller, J. T., Wiss, A. L., May, C. C., Jones, G. M., & Smetana, K. S. (2019, April/June). Acute management of hypertension following intracerebral hemorrhage. *Critical Care Nursing Quarterly, 42*(2), 129–147. https://doi.org/10.1097/CNQ.0000000000000247

Hikma Pharmaceuticals USA, Inc. (2020). *Hydralazine hydrochloride injection*. https://dailymed.nlm.nih.gov/dailymed/fda/fdaDrugXsl.cfm?setid=3f5f1204-d289-40e9-be84-a29352f64bfb&type=display

Laurent, S. (2017). Antihypertensive drugs. *Pharmacological Research, 124*, 116–125. https://doi.org/10.1016/j.phrs.2017.07.026

Powers, W. J., Rabinstein, A. A., Ackerson, T., Adeoye, O. M., Bambakidis, N. C., Becker, K., Biller, J., Brown, M., Demaerschalk, B. M., Hoh, B., Jauch, E. C., Kidwell, C. S., Leslie-Mazwi, T. M., Ovbiagele, B., Scott, P. A., Sheth, K. N., Southerland, A. M., Summers, D. V., & Tirschwell, D. L. (2019). Guidelines for the early management of patients with acute ischemic stroke: 2019 update to the 2018 guidelines for the early management of acute ischemic stroke: A guideline for healthcare professionals from the American Heart Association/American Stroke Association. *Stroke, 50*(12), e344–e418. https://doi.org/10.1161/STR.0000000000000211

Precision Dose, Inc. (2017). *Phentolamine mesylate*. https://dailymed.nlm.nih.gov/dailymed/fda/fdaDrugXsl.cfm?setid=e146c7ee-d2fa-433c-8768-0945e4ff0990&type=display

Smetana, K. S., Buschur, P. L., Owusu-Guha, J., & May, C. C. (2020). Pharmacologic management of cerebral vasospasm in aneurysmal subarachnoid hemorrhage. *Critical Care Nursing Quarterly, 43*(2), 138–156. https://doi.org/10.1097/CNQ.0000000000000299

Teligent Pharma, Inc. (2018). *Vitamin K*. https://www.accessdata.fda.gov/drugsatfda_docs/label/2018/012223s042lbl.pdf

West-Ward Pharmaceutical Corp. (2010). *Enalaprilat*. https://dailymed.nlm.nih.gov/dailymed/fda/fdaDrugXsl.cfm?setid=eabae489-e254-4987-ab90-7cda20a6f856&type=display

Xiromed, LLC. (2021). *Sodium nitroprusside*. https://dailymed.nlm.nih.gov/dailymed/fda/fdaDrugXsl.cfm?setid=90f4f18f-eb6a-d700-6ec4-c4961f6ab49c&type=display#CLINICAL_PHARMACOLOGY

11

Stroke Unit Care

Brittney Bradshaw

The stroke unit is a unique environment equipped to take stroke patients directly from the emergency room or from the intensive care unit. Thus, much of the initial care is similar to what is described elsewhere. Some parts of stroke care are unique to the stroke care unit, as it finishes the stroke workup and gets the patient ready for discharge.

STROKE UNIT CARE

Noninterventional Acute Stroke Care

Admission to a Specialized Stroke Unit

- Designation for a primary stroke center entails that the facility must have a specified stroke unit.
- Dedicated stroke units provide an interdisciplinary team of specially trained nurses, physicians, therapists, and social worker personnel.
- Pathways and processes put into place by these units have been proven to decrease the likelihood of death, disability, and dependence at one-year poststroke, as well as reduce medical complications and improve outcomes.

Antiplatelets

- For patients with noncardioembolic ischemic stroke or transient ischemic attack (TIA), antiplatelets are preferred over anticoagulation in reducing risk of recurrent stroke. In those with allergies to aspirin, monotherapy with clopidogrel (Plavix) is a safe alternative. If the patient is a P2Y12 nonresponder, alternative antiplatelet therapy, such as ticagrelor (Brilinta), can be used.

Blood Pressure Management

- Profound hypertension (HTN) and hypotension have been linked to poor outcomes.

- Cerebral autoregulation may be absent in the acute phase of stroke, leaving the brain even more vulnerable to extremes of blood pressure (BP).
- Elevation of BP during an acute stroke can be a compensatory mechanism to raise cerebral perfusion and amplify collateral circulation.
- While the exact BP goal for the acute phase of ischemic stroke is unknown, it is acceptable to gradually reduce BP by 15% over 24 hours, while maintaining a minimum systolic blood pressure (SBP) of 150.
- Exceptions to this rule include those patients who need BP control, including those with an aortic dissection or myocardial infarction, and so forth.
- Hypotension should be avoided, and when observed, an underlying cause should be investigated and treated. Prolonged chair sitting should be avoided.
- Safety in provoking HTN through vasopressors has not been shown in large trials, however permissive and induced HTN may benefit some select patients. Patients should be observed for side effects of vasopressors and volume expanders such as cardiac ischemia and fluid overload.

Statins

- High-intensity statin should be initiated for those with ischemic stroke or TIA, which further reduces risk of stroke and cardiovascular events
- Goal low-density lipoprotein (LDL) long-term of <70 mg/dL

STROKE COMPLICATIONS

Hyperglycemia and Hypoglycemia

- Hyperglycemia is common after a stroke and may be a culmination of a stress response, diabetes, or impaired glucose tolerance.
- Hyperglycemia has been linked to poorer outcomes in stroke (long-term mortality and decreased functional capacity), however aggressive hyperglycemia treatment measurements may not be favorable, as they cause hypoglycemia in 15% to 35% of those patients that are aggressively treated.
- Hypoglycemia should be avoided and should be treated if glucose <70 mg/dL.
- Target glucose levels following a stroke, during hospital admission, is 140 to 180 mg/dL.
- Hemoglobin A1c (Hgb A1c) should be performed on admission, with long-term goal Hgb A1c of <7.0.

FAST FACTS

Hypoglycemia can mimic stroke and should be one of the first things checked in a patient with an acute change of mental status.

Dysphagia and Nutrition

- All stroke patients should be screened for dysphagia within the first 24 hours of presentation (Lee et al., 2012).

- The patient should have nothing by mouth (NPO) until their ability to swallow has been tested.
- A validated screening tool should be utilized to assess for dysphagia, and if dysphagia is suspected through the screening tool or based on clinical presentation, the patient should remain NPO.
- It is important to keep in mind that stroke patients can experience silent aspiration without outward signs of difficulty swallowing, such as coughing.
- Speech and language pathologists (SLPs) should be consulted in those with suspected dysphagia, and video fluoroscopic swallow studies may be performed.
- Nasogastric (NG) tubes on the stroke unit are not recommended for use until a formal evaluation can take place. Stroke center standards indicate that once ordered, the evaluation should take place within 24 hours. NG tubes are recommended if the patient is unable to meet nutritional needs orally or requires critical medications that cannot be safely administered without enteral access.

Gastrointestinal Bleeding

- Use of H2 blockers, proton pump inhibitors, or sucralfate can aid in preventing gastrointestinal (GI) bleeding, however H2 blockers and proton pump inhibitors are associated with an increased risk of pneumonia.
- Routine administration of peptic ulcer prophylaxis is not recommended in the stroke population as the risk of peptic ulcers is relatively low.
- Risk factors of developing a GI bleed include severe stroke, cancer, sepsis, peptic ulcer disease, abnormal liver function, renal failure, anticoagulation, and feeding through an NG tube.
- When a GI bleed occurs, antithrombotic medications are often stopped, which may increase risk for recurrent strokes, myocardial infarctions, and venous thromboembolism.

Hyperthermia and Infections

- Hyperthermia has been associated with poorer outcomes in those with ischemic and hemorrhagic stroke.
- Stroke patients (both hemorrhagic and ischemic) can have a central fever, which is a spontaneous increase in temperature that is not associated with an infection but is related to an inflammatory response from damage to the thermoregulatory system (pons and hypothalamus) or from blood in the intraventricular space.
- Antipyretic agents such as acetaminophen or ibuprofen are commonly used to control fever.
- Endovascular or surface cooling are also effective in reducing fever, but shivering should be avoided.
- Infectious causes of fever should be investigated and treated: bacteremia, pneumonia, urinary tract infection, and decubitus ulcers.
- The most common cause of pneumonia in a stroke patient is aspiration, which can cause gastric contents aspiration (chemical pneumonitis) and/or an infectious pneumonia from pharyngeal flora.

- Risk factors of pneumonia include being an older adult, cognitive impairment, severe facial palsy, disabling stroke, brainstem stroke, multiple territory stroke, mechanical ventilation, weakened cough from expiratory/pharyngeal muscle weakness, and decreased level of consciousness.
- Prevention of aspiration pneumonia includes dysphagia screening, frequent oral care, and semi-upright positioning.
- Supplemental oxygen should be utilized to maintain an oxygen saturation of >94%.
- Mobilization and sitting up in a chair should be encouraged as appropriate to augment lung expansion.
- Urinary tract infection (UTI) risk factors include being an older adult, female gender, disabling stroke, and indwelling urinary catheters. Risk may be reduced by removing and avoiding indwelling catheters, as well as ensuring adequate fluid intake.
- Decubitus ulcers can result from immobilization, fecal incontinence, and urinary incontinence.
- Prevention of decubitus ulcers includes regular examination in bedridden patients, early and frequent mobilization, frequent every 2-hour turning and cleaning, air mattresses, and padded heel supports.

Deep Vein Thrombosis and Pulmonary Embolism

- Risk factors for deep vein thrombosis (DVT) include being an older adult, immobility, and dehydration.
- Untreated DVT can lead to a pulmonary embolism (PE) and is a considerable cause of death in stroke patients.
- Routine screenings for DVT's without accompanying symptoms are not typically recommended but may be appropriate for those with lower extremity swelling, lower extremity pain, low-grade unexplained fevers, or unexplained elevated white blood cell counts.
- Mechanical (pneumatic compression devices) or pharmacological prophylaxis (Heparin or Lovenox subcutaneously) should be initiated in nonambulatory stroke patients. Thromboembolic deterrent (TED) stockings are not recommended in the acute setting.
- Range of motion (ROM) exercises and stretching of the paretic limb should be done while nonambulatory.
- Encouragement and support for ambulation—when permitted—is beneficial in prevention.

FAST FACTS

One rule of thumb is that patients should continue to receive both pharmacologic and mechanical DVT prophylaxis until the patient is able to independently walk to the bathroom.

CARDIAC COMPLICATIONS

- Ischemic stroke patients should be screened for abnormal cardiac biomarkers such as an elevated troponin level, have a baseline EKG, and have an echocardiogram performed.
- Continuous cardiac monitoring is recommended for at least 24 to 48 hours after a stroke to evaluate for arrhythmias, such as atrial fibrillation, that could have contributed to the stroke.
- Risk factors for developing arrhythmias include prolonged QT interval seen on echocardiogram or strokes involving the right insula.
- Patients with diabetes, peripheral artery disease, coronary artery disease, and large strokes are at elevated risk for cardiac complications.
- Cardiac biomarkers may be elevated due to a stress response following stroke or from autonomic dysfunction (strokes involving the right insula).
- Patients with large artery-related strokes are at higher risk for myocardial infarction.
- Takotsubo cardiomyopathy, also known as "stunned myocardium" or "broken heart syndrome," can occur in patients within 24 hours of stroke and can be seen with "apical ballooning" or ST elevation seen on EKG.
- Acute myocardial infarction (MI), volume overload, and neurogenic causes can contribute to the development of congestive heart failure.

Pain

- Evaluating and treating pain in stroke patients is vital.
- Pain is relatively rare in stroke patients, largely being headache, shoulder pain, or decubitus ulcer, if present.
- Patients with immobile limbs can have pain from positioning or from spasming associated with the weight of the limb.
- Thalamic pain syndrome, now called central poststroke pain, can occur in those with a stroke (hemorrhagic or ischemic) involving their thalamus. This is a neuropathic pain syndrome and is associated with temperature changes. Deficits in thermoregulation occur due to damage in the spinothalamic tract. This pain syndrome can occur acutely after stroke, in the subacute period, or years following the stroke (Dydyk & Munakomi, 2022).
- Pharmacological and nonpharmacological measures should be implemented to treat pain.

Constipation

- Dehydration, decreased mobility, and opioid use following stroke contribute to constipation.
- Bowel function, bowel habits, bowel sounds, and abdominal distention should all be evaluated.
- A bowel regimen with stool softeners, laxatives, and enemas may be required to prevent constipation and/or ileus.
- Encouragement and support for ambulation—when permitted—is beneficial.

Urinary Dysfunction

- Urinary incontinence is a widespread problem following a stroke.
- Additionally, stroke patients are at risk for urinary retention, hyperreflexia, neurogenic bladder, urge incontinence, and overflow incontinence.
- Stroke patients may require bladder scanning and straight catheterization every 4 to 6 hours.
- Bladder retraining with offering urinal, bedpan, commode every 2 hours while awake and every 4 hours at night is beneficial; in addition, limiting fluid intake in the evening may be helpful.

Seizures

- Poststroke epilepsy is common as there is neuronal dysfunction as a result of ischemic tissue both from hemorrhagic or ischemic stroke beds.
- In the acute phase of stroke, seizure is caused by edema or presence of intraparenchymal blood. However, seizure is less common in the acute phase and does not warrant preventative use of antiepileptics.
- In the chronic phase of stroke, scar tissue and neuronal deformities can cause seizure.

Depression

- Depression is common after acute stroke and can inhibit participation in therapy and communication with others.
- Regular assessment of mood is beneficial in detection of early signs of depression.
- If noted, antidepressants should be considered and discussed with the patient and family.

EARLY THERAPY EVALUATION

- Early mobilization and rehabilitation offer patients their best opportunity for recovery following a stroke (Livesay et al., 2014).
- A patient's functional and cognitive abilities should be assessed by physical therapy and occupational therapy (Teasell et al., 2020).

Family Involvement

- Daily team rounds should include a family member whenever possible.
  - Ensures that family is aware of current plan of care, as stroke patients may have cognitive or communication deficits
  - Facilitates realistic discharge plans
  - Enables family to participate in plan of care, as well as assisting with passive exercises, mobilization, and feeding

TOAST CRITERIA

The Trial of Org 10172 in Acute Stroke Treatment (TOAST) is a system used to classify ischemic strokes into five different subtypes: large-artery atherosclerosis (LAA), cardioembolism (CE), small-artery occlusion/lacune (SAO), stroke of other determined etiology (rare causes), and stroke of undetermined etiology (cryptogenic). Stroke management, prognosis, and risk of recurrence are all shaped by the stroke subtypes. These causes of ischemic stroke are identified through tests such as brain/vessel imaging (CT/MRI), cardiac imaging (echocardiography, etc.), duplex imaging of extracranial arteries, and labs assessing coagulopathy/autoimmune states (Adams et al., 1993).

LARGE ARTERY ATHEROSCLEROSIS

LAA is the cause of about 15% of all ischemic strokes. Patients will have >50% stenosis or occlusion of major extracranial (carotid disease) or intracranial arteries. These lesions can be divided into four categories: asymptomatic and symptomatic extracranial carotid stenosis, extracranial vertebral artery atherosclerosis, and intracranial atherosclerosis (ICAS). The LAA lesion should be close to the vascular region supplying the patient's stroke area, or clinical symptoms should correlate in the setting of TIA (Chaturvedi & Bhattacharya, 2014).

Imaging Used to Confirm Diagnosis

- Arteriographic studies through CT or MRI (CT angiogram [CTA] brain/neck or magnetic resonance angiogram [MRA] brain/neck)
- Cerebral angiogram
- Carotid duplex

Medical Management

- Intensive medical therapy: antiplatelets (mono vs. dual), intensive lipid-lowering agents (not just targeting for a specific level of LDL), long-term BP management includes identifying physiologic causes of resistant HTN; plasma renin and aldosterone levels, diabetes management by referring to endocrinology if Hgb A1c uncontrolled despite medical therapy, smoking cessation, diet, and exercise (Cole, 2017)
- Intracranial atherosclerosis:
  - SAMPRISS trial delved into safety/efficacy of percutaneous transluminal angioplasty and stenting (PTAS) with aggressive medical management versus medical management in patients with recent stroke or TIA (within 30 days) due to 70% to 99% stenosis of a crucial intracranial artery. Medical management included 325 mg of aspirin daily and Plavix 75 mg daily for 90 days. Medical management was superior to PTAS with medical management in preventing recurrence of stroke (Chimowitz et al., 2011).
- Permissive HTN to avoid hypoperfusion and furthering stroke burden; allow time to develop improved collateral circulation

Carotid Artery Stenting Versus Carotid Endarterectomy

- Carotid revascularization within 2 weeks of stroke or TIA is preferred over delaying for 6 weeks or more.
- Carotid endarterectomy (CEA) removes carotid artery plaque through an open surgical technique. CEA is usually the treatment choice for those who have 70% or more of carotid artery stenosis and are symptomatic.

- There is a higher complication rate (MI, stroke, and death) in patients older than 70 years who get carotid artery stenting (CAS) versus CEA; however, this procedure may be appropriate for certain patients with advanced age or other perioperative risk factors that may favor stenting.
- For more information, see Chapter 8 on endovascular and surgical management.

CARDIOEMBOLISM

Cardioembolic (CE) strokes are due to an embolism arising from the heart. Around 29% of ischemic strokes are of cardiac origin. Involvement of more than one vascular region and findings of systemic embolism support a cardiogenic cause of stroke. A CE etiology of stroke is often examined if there is nonlacunar stroke, and the patient is without intracranial artery disease in the setting of numerous strokes. Frequent causes of CE stroke are coronary artery disease, atrial fibrillation, valvular heart disease, mitral calcification, and cardiomyopathy. Some high-risk sources of CE stroke include mechanical prosthetic valves, atrial fibrillation, left atrial appendage thrombus, dilated cardiomyopathy, atrial myxoma (tumor), and infective endocarditis. Some medium-risk sources of CE stroke include atrial septal aneurysm, patent foramen ovale (PFO), nonbacterial thrombotic endocarditis, and myocardial infarct.

Imaging and Diagnostics Used to Confirm Diagnosis

- Transthoracic echocardiogram (TTE) and transesophageal echocardiogram (TEE) are utilized to evaluate cardiac thrombus, valvular abnormalities, or evidence of a PFO.
- TTE provides limited visualization of the left atrial appendage and left atrium due to anatomical location. TEE provides better visualization of cardiac anatomy and identification of an embolic source of stroke.
- Cardiac MRI or cardiac CT can also identify valvular causes of stroke.
- In evaluating underlying arrhythmias such as atrial fibrillation as the cause of stroke, a 30-day cardiac telemetry monitor can help detect paroxysmal and persistent atrial fibrillation. Implantable rhythm recording devices (LOOP or LINQ) can provide long-term monitoring for arrhythmias. Prolonged EKG monitoring can also assist in detecting atrial fibrillation.

Medical Management

- In patients with CE source of stroke, anticoagulation is superior in preventing stroke as opposed to antiplatelets.
- However, in those with infective endocarditis, prior to initiating anticoagulation, the patient may warrant a direct cerebral angiography to evaluate for the presence of mycotic aneurysms, as they can cause intracerebral hemorrhage. The mainstay of medical treatment for infective endocarditis is antibiotic therapy, and infectious disease should be on board.

- The ideal timing for beginning anticoagulation in those without large strokes or uncontrolled HTN is within 2 weeks of a stroke or TIA.
- In atrial fibrillation, rhythm control is superior to rate reduction in preventing future strokes.

Surgical Management

- In those with cardiac myxomas, surgical resection should be considered to prevent future recurrent stroke.
- In those with endocarditis, a valve replacement may be warranted, and the patient should be evaluated by cardiothoracic surgery.

SMALL-ARTERY OCCLUSION

SAOs are subcortical infarcts that result from occlusion of a single penetrating artery also known as lacunar infarcts and are typically <15 mm in diameter. Common locations of lacunar infarcts are basal ganglia (caudate, thalamus, globus pallidus, and putamen), subcortical white matter (internal capsule and corona radiata), cerebellum, and pons.

Imaging and Diagnostics Used to Confirm Diagnosis

- CT of the brain or MRI of the brain will confirm location and size of the stroke (Mendelson & Prabhakaran, 2021).
- CTA, MRA, or a vascular duplex of the carotid arteries confirms the absence of intracranial/extracranial atherosclerosis as the cause of stroke.
- Along with the imaging, location, and size of the stroke, a TTE and echocardiogram can be used to evaluate the absence of cardiac causes of stroke.

Medical Management

- Medical management consists of intensive medical therapy with antiplatelets (mono vs. dual), intensive lipid-lowering agents, long-term BP management, diabetes management, smoking cessation, diet, and exercise.

STROKE OF ANOTHER DETERMINED CAUSE

These causes of stroke are rare and only account for around 5% of strokes. These causes are broken down into several categories: infectious, hematologic abnormalities, inflammatory conditions, noninflammatory conditions of the arterial wall, and hereditary conditions.

Infections

- **Bacterial:** meningitis from *Streptococcus pneumoniae, Neisseria meningitides, Hemophilus influenzae*, tuberculous meningitis, and meningovascular syphilis
- **Viral:** herpes zoster (particularly opthalmicus), HIV vasculopathy
- **Fungal:** aspergillus, rhinocerebral mucormycosis
- **Parasitic:** neurocysticercosis, Chagas disease

Hematologic

- **White blood cell causes:** leukemia and intravascular lymphoma
- **Hyperviscosity syndromes:** Waldenstrom's macroglobulinemia, chylomicra, and multiple myeloma
- **Red blood cell causes:** sickle cell anemia, polycythemia vera
- **Platelet causes**: thrombocytosis, sticky platelet syndrome
- **Clotting factor/hypercoagulability:** certain chemotherapy agents, Trousseau syndrome, pregnancy, oral contraceptive and hormone therapy, thrombotic thrombocytopenic purpura, disseminated intravascular coagulation, oral contraceptives and hormone therapy, heparin-induced thrombocytopenia with thrombosis, inflammatory bowel disease, polycystic kidney disease, and marantic endocarditis

Inflammatory

- **Causes**: primary central nervous system and systemic vasculitis, systemic lupus erythematosus, rheumatoid arthritis, Behcet's disease, and sarcoidosis

Noninflammatory Conditions of the Arterial Wall

- **Causes**: moyamoya disease, cervicocephalic arterial dissections, and fibromuscular dysplasia

Hereditary

- **Small vessel causes:** Fabry disease, cerebral autosomal dominant arteriopathy with subcortical infarcts and leukoencephalopathy, cerebral autosomal recessive arteriopathy with subcortical infarcts and leukoencephalopathy, retinal vasculopathy with cerebral leukodystrophy
- **Connective tissue disorders:** Marfan syndrome, Ehlers-Danlos syndrome, osteogenesis imperfectica, and Pseudoxanthoma elasticum
- **Mitochondrial disorders:** mitochondrial myopathy, encephalopathy, lactic acidosis, and stroke-like symptoms (MELAS) and myoclonic epilepsy with ragged red ribers (MERRF)

STROKE OF UNDETERMINED CAUSE (CRYPTOGENIC)

Around 40% of strokes can be attributed to an undetermined cause. A cryptogenic stroke is when the cause of the stroke has not been identified despite comprehensive evaluation for potential causes of stroke (definite CE, LAA, or SAO), which includes utilizing cardiac, vascular, and serological workup of stroke.

Imaging Used to Confirm Diagnosis

- CT or MRI of the brain will confirm location and size of the stroke.
- CT or MR angiography, or a vascular duplex of the carotid arteries, confirms the absence of intracranial/extracranial atherosclerosis as the cause of stroke.
- Along with the imaging, location, and size of the stroke, a TTE and echocardiogram can be used to confirm the absence of cardiac causes of stroke.

Medical Management

- Antiplatelet therapy is superior to empiric anticoagulation.
- Minimizing risk factors that cause stroke: HTN, smoking, hyperlipidemia, and so forth

Additional Diagnoses

- Implantable rhythm recording devices (LOOP or LINQ) can provide long-term monitoring for arrhythmias as up to 23% of patients with cryptogenic stroke have paroxysmal atrial fibrillation.
- Especially in those less than 45 years old without risk factors, laboratory tests to detect hypercoagulable states that could contribute to cryptogenic stroke should be obtained. These include B-2 glycoprotein, fibrinogen, homocysteine lipoprotein "A," C-reactive protein, prothrombin gene, cardiolipin Ab, Factor V Leiden, methyl tetrahydrofolate (MTHFR) mutation analysis, protein C, protein S, antithrombin III, lupus anticoagulant, Factor VIII, and hemoglobin electrophoresis.
- Consider recommending cessation of oral contraceptives and testosterone therapy in cryptogenic stroke in the young.
- In the presence of PFO, lower extremity dopplers can be obtained to evaluate for venous thrombosis.
- Consider performing a lumbar puncture to rule out vasculitis.

HEMORRHAGIC STROKE

Intracranial Hemorrhage

Intracranial hemorrhage (ICH) is the second most common type of stroke. ICH is more common in those older than 55 years of age and more common in men than women. The primary goal of treating ICH is to restrict hematoma extension. Other goals are to prevent elevated intracranial pressure, herniation, and seizures.

Etiology

Hypertension

- HTN is the main risk factor for developing a spontaneous ICH. Increased risk of developing ICH is in patients who smoke, are 55 years or older, and are noncompliant with their antihypertensive regimen. Common locations for hypertensive-related ICH are the thalamus, basal ganglia, cerebral lobes, pons, and cerebellum.

Cerebral Amyloid Angiopathy

- Cerebral amyloid angiopathy (CAA) is distinguished by beta amyloid protein deposits in the leptomeninges and cerebral cortex blood vessels. This can cause lobar ICH in patients older than 60 years of age.

Vascular Malformation

- Arteriovenous malformation (AVM), cavernous malformations, and angiomas can cause ICH and should be considered if there is a lobar hemorrhage in a young individual without a history of HTN. After the initial hemorrhagic event, AVMs can be visualized with a CT angiogram or a direct cerebral angiogram (DCA).

Venous Sinus Thrombosis

- Cerebral venous sinus thrombosis is a rare cause of ICH, but primarily affects middle aged females. Risk factors for venous sinus thrombosis are hypercoagulable states, local infections (otitis, sinusitis, and mastoiditis), and inflammatory disorders. Magnetic resonance venogram, CT venogram, and DCA can evaluate for venous sinus thrombosis. Patients treated with heparin to prevent clot extension have improved outcomes, even though there is risk for hematoma expansion.

Other

- Other causes of ICH to consider are anticoagulation (warfarin or direct-thrombin inhibitors), fibrinolytic therapy, coagulopathy (impaired clotting function due to hemophilia, platelet dysfunction, liver dysfunction, uremia, etc.), excessive alcohol use, vasculitis, sympathomimetic drugs (cocaine, methamphetamine, pseudoephedrine, phenylpropanolamine), primary intracranial tumors, and metastatic tumors.

SUBARACHNOID HEMORRHAGE

Most spontaneous subarachnoid hemorrhages (SAHs) are from cerebral aneurysms. Aneurysmal SAHs are either surgically clipped or coiled to stop bleeding. Other causes of spontaneous SAH include intracranial dissection, AVMs, and angiographic negative SAH (with perimesencephalic hemorrhage).

Imaging

- A CT of the head is sensitive to detecting an acute hemorrhage and should be repeated 6 hours after initial presentation to evaluate for hematoma expansion. MRI is most sensitive for recognizing a previous hemorrhage. CT angiography and CT head with contrast are useful in evaluating those at elevated risk of hematoma expansion in the setting of contrast extravasation within the hematoma "the spot sign."

Medical Management

- Medical management consists of intensive medical therapy with long-term BP management, diabetes management, smoking cessation, diet, and exercise.
- Additional acute management can be found in Chapter 9, ICU Stroke Care.
- Secondary prevention management can be found in Chapter 14, Primary and Secondary Stroke Prevention.

References

Adams, Jr. H. P., Bendixen, B. H., Kappelle, L. J., Biller, J., Love, B. B., Gordon, D. L., & Marsh, III E. E. (1993, January). Classification of subtype of acute ischemic stroke.

Definitions for use in a multicenter clinical trial. TOAST. Trial of Org 10172 in acute stroke treatment. *Stroke, 24*(1), 35–41. https://doi.org/10.1161/01.str.24.1.35

Chaturvedi, S., & Bhattacharya, P. (2014, April). Large artery atherosclerosis: Carotid stenosis, vertebral artery disease, and intracranial atherosclerosis. *Continuum (Minneap Minn), 20*(2 Cerebrovascular Disease), 323–334. https://doi.org/10.1212/01.CON.0000446104.90043.a5

Chimowitz, M. I., Lynn, M. J., Derdeyn, C. P., Turan, T. N., Fiorella, D., Lane, B. F., Scott Janis, L., Lutsep, H. L., Barnwell, S. L., Waters, M. F., Hoh, B. L., Hourihane, J. M., Levy, E. I., Alexandrov, A. V., Harrigan, M. R., Chiu, D., Klucznik, R. P., Clark, J. M., McDougall, C. G., ... Cloft, H. J. (2011). Stenting versus aggressive medical therapy for intracranial arterial stenosis. *New England Journal of Medicine, 365*(11), 993–1003.

Cole, J. W. (2017, February). Large artery atherosclerotic occlusive disease. *Continuum, 23*(1, Cerebrovascular Disease), 133–157. https://doi.org/10.1212/CON.0000000000000436

Dydyk, A. M., & Munakomi, S. (2022, January). *Thalamic pain syndrome*. StatPearls Publishing. https://www.ncbi.nlm.nih.gov/books/NBK554490/

Lee, V. H., Lazzaro, M., Prabhakaran, S., Connors, J., Rosenberg, N., John, S., Garg, R., & Temes, R. (2012). *Handbook of stroke and neurocritical care* (pp. 23–213). Essay, Nova Science Publishers.

Livesay, S., Wilson, S., Baumann, J. J., Hepburn, M., Brophy, G., Castle, A., Neyens, R., Szabo, C., Higgins, P. G., Straw, M., Kelly, M., & American Association of Neuroscience Nurses. (2014). AANN *comprehensive review for stroke nursing*. American Association of Neuroscience Nurses.

Mendelson, S. J., & Prabhakaran, S. (2021, March 16). Diagnosis and management of transient ischemic attack and acute ischemic stroke: A review. *JAMA, 325*(11), 1088–1098. https://doi.org/10.1001/jama.2020.26867

Teasell, R., Salbach, N. M., Foley, N., Mountain, A., Cameron, J. I., Jong, A., Acerra, N. E., Bastasi, D., Carter, S. L., Fung, J., Halabi, M. L., Iruthayarajah, J., Harris, J., Kim, E., Noland, A., Pooyania, S., Rochette, A., Stack, B. D., Symcox, E., Timpson, D., Varghese, S., Verrilli, S., Gubitz, G., Casaubon, L. K., Dowlatshahi, D., & Lindsay, M. P. (2020, October). Canadian stroke best practice recommendations: Rehabilitation, recovery, and community participation following stroke. Part one: Rehabilitation and recovery following stroke; 6th edition update 2019. *International Journal of Stroke, 15*(7), 763–788. Epub 2020 January 27. https://doi.org/10.1177/1747493019897843

12

Telestroke

Randheer Yadav and Noah Grose

Efforts have been made to reduce the time from identification of possible stroke to evaluation and treatment. Early thrombolysis therapy is clinically effective in reducing neurological deficits and disability. Only a small fraction of acute stroke patients were being treated with IV thrombolytic therapy at small and community hospitals due to unavailability of experts in acute stroke care. Transferring these patients to a hospital capable of providing treatments for acute stroke may take several minutes to hours making many of these patients ineligible to receive acute stroke therapies leading to worse clinical outcomes. Expecting every community hospital to have experts in acute stroke care is not fiscally feasible nor sustainable. Technological advancements such as telemedicine have provided a solution to this barrier in the field of medicine.

FAST FACTS

Risk factors for stroke are more prevalent, and specialized stroke treatment options are less available in rural and remote areas. Only 2% to 4% of ischemic stroke patients receive IV thrombolytic therapy with the lowest percentage in rural areas.

TELEMEDICINE/TELEHEALTH

Telemedicine or telehealth is the provision of healthcare remotely by utilizing telecommunication technologies. It allows long-distance patient and clinician contact for history, physical examination, and intervention. In its simple form, telehealth may involve communication between clinician and the patient via telephone audio only, and in its more sophisticated form it may involve interactive physical examination on video and remote surgeries. When this concept is used in providing care to stroke patients, it is commonly referred to as telestroke.

- Some form of telemedicine existed in the 19th century. Telegraphy communicated information about medical supplies and casualty lists concerning U.S. Civil War victims.
- Telestroke originated in the late 1980s and 1990s.
- TeleBAT was one of the earliest programs implemented at the University of Maryland to transmit information from emergency medical services (EMS) to the receiving hospital.

TELESTROKE

Telestroke allows delivery of live two-way vascular neuroscience consultations using a telecommunications infrastructure. Telestroke enables proper triage and guidance by distant specialists, remote imaging assessment, teleconsultation, and remote thrombolysis which increases treatment rates and decreases treatment times (Tumma et al., 2022). A mobile stroke unit is one way of implementing the telestroke strategy which involves the concept of bringing the hospital to the patient. Another concept is a hub-and-spoke hospital network which brings specialized care to nonspecialized hospitals.

A systematic review of 19 studies involving 28,496 subjects comprising prehospital and in-hospital telestroke interventions shows the benefits of telestroke:

- Increased odds of successful treatment of patients within 3 hours by twofold
- Improved outcomes at 3 months
- Shorter onset to treatment times
- Lower in-hospital mortality rates

Models have been developed to compare and analyze the cost-effectiveness of the telestroke networks. These models conclude that hub-and-spoke telestroke networks are cost effective (Nelson et al., 2011). One such model looking at a network of one hub and seven spokes predicts:

- Telestroke networks may result in annual cost savings of $358,435.
- Telestroke networks may result in more IV thrombolysis, more endovascular stroke therapies, more stroke patients discharged home independently, and so, greater cost savings for the entire network.
- Hospital costs are associated with transfer rate. Higher patient transfer rates diminish the cost savings for the spoke hospitals.

Another such model used a decision-analytic model to study 90-day and lifetime horizons. Quality-adjusted life-years (QALYs) gained were combined with costs to generate incremental cost-effectiveness ratios (ICERs).

- Over a lifetime, telestroke is cost-effective compared to usual care. Telestroke costs are upfront, but the benefits of improved stroke care are lifelong.
- Compared to usual care, telestroke results in an ICER of $2,449/QALY in the lifetime horizon.

Telestroke Advantages

Telestroke has been beneficial for individuals and communities in receiving specialized stroke care regardless of geographic location (Lazarus et al., 2020). Telestroke has been an equally beneficial model of care for hospital systems.

- Telestroke providesacute stroke care access to a larger population (only 64% of the U.S. population lives witin 60 minutes' driving distance of a comprehensive or thrombectomy capable stroke center).
- In 2019, of the 5,587 EDs in the United States, 2,505 (45%) were categorized as having telestroke services (Zachrison et al., 2022).
- Telestroke enables delivery of specialized care at nonspecialized hospitals.
- Telestroke allows quick and accurate treatment decision-making for acute stroke patients.
- Telestroke helps significantly reduce the onset of symptoms to treatment time.
- It compensates for the lack of neurologists and human resources.
- It helps decrease geographic disparities of acute stroke care.
- Telestroke is a cost-effective method of delivering acute stroke care to communities without access to on-site stroke specialists.
- Telestroke supports follow-up compliance for patients with barriers such as distance or lack of transportation.

Telestroke Setup

Initial setup of telestroke systems of care requires much discussion, planning, and development of continued methods for quality assessment and improvement.

- Extensive planning with key stakeholders and multidisciplinary involvement
- Standardized protocols and procedures
- Necessary equipment and adequate staffing
- Stakeholder engagement and training
- Availability for technical assistance for reliable services

Telestroke Challenges/Considerations

As telestroke systems of care involve clients, staffing, infrastructure development, and technology, the challenges are also multifactorial:

- Space implications for hardware in emergency department
- Software and hardware integration with the provider system including imaging software
- Quick and reliable technical support
- Additional staff availability
- Sustainability in spoke sites with low stroke volumes
- Confidentiality and privacy: These have been areas of concern in healthcare, but telemedicine presents even greater challenges in maintaining confidentiality and privacy of the patients.

ADVANCES IN TELEMEDICINE

Telemedicine principles of care are no different, but the method of delivery is different. Telemedicine systems of care have seen many changes since they were initially used. These changes have been in different dimensions.

- Technological and infrastructure advancements
  Remote and rural areas often lack infrastructure, but a bigger challenge is the availability of a reliable network. While 30 to 40 years ago communication was more dependent on landline phones and faxes, we now have much

wider availability of faster networks that enable real-time audio and video two-way communication.
  - The advances have been qualitative as well as geographic in that such facilities are now available in a majority of rural areas.
  - Advancements allow for uninterrupted telestroke visits and minimize frustration to both patients and clinicians.

- Regulatory advancements
  As mentioned in the challenges of telemedicine, confidentiality and privacy of patients have been a priority in healthcare. Telemedicine presents a greater risk to confidentiality and privacy as it involves two different geographic locations and more channels of information sharing.
  - The Department of Health and Human Services and other agencies provide guidance for clinicians as well as education for the public on measures to maintain privacy and confidentiality for telemedicine visit.
  - Guidelines for credentialing clinicians have been developed at both the hub and the spoke hospitals.
  - Documentation of visit and information sharing practices among the stakeholders have improved.

BILLING FOR TELEHEALTH SERVICES

Some of the most complicated challenges to the development of telehealth have been related to billing practices.

- Questions regarding compensation in comparison to in-person visit.
- Differences in payer rules for reimbursement continue to be resolved: Centers for Medicare & Medicaid Services pays nurse practitioner services at 80% of the lesser of the actual charge or 85% of the amount a physician gets under the Medicare Physician Fee Schedule.
- Clinicians and billers continue to learn best practices for submitting the appropriate bills.

CLINICIANS AND USER EXPERIENCES

Both clinicians and patients have grown in their experiences with the use of telemedicine.

- Clinicians have become much more proficient in utilizing technologies and applications.
- Community awareness and patients' experiences regarding telehealth have grown.

CURRENT STATE

The COVID-19 pandemic and telestroke (and telehealth in general) have tremendously helped each other. Telemedicine as a discipline was getting momentum even in the years prior to the pandemic, but the pandemic helped telemedicine move fast forward. Telemedicine has been included in the acute ischemic stroke guidelines from the American Heart Association and American Stroke Association.

- Administration of IV thrombolysis by utilizing teleradiology and telestroke can be effective for correct decision-making.
- Telestroke networks can be helpful in triaging patients with acute ischemic stroke who may be considered mechanical thrombectomy.
- The COVID-19 pandemic ensured that telehealth was utilized in every aspect of healthcare and in every specialty.

FUTURE TRENDS

As telestroke networks become more proficient in technological, practical, regulatory, and billing aspects, various other dimensions are being explored. One possibility is keeping stroke patients at the spoke hospital if they don't need any acute stroke therapy.

- Telestroke network size and utilization have increased over time.
- Patients who are ineligible for advanced stroke therapy are staying at spoke hospitals for completion of their stroke workup.
- Telestroke services are being expanded to provide follow-up services after the acute stroke visit.
- Advanced practice providers (APPs) are playing a larger role in providing telestroke services where no neurovascular expertise is available.
- CMS and other payers continue to review their guidelines to appropriately reimburse for the services provided using telestroke networks.
- Representation of APPs in telestroke networks of care continues to grow.
- Efforts for reasonable compensation to APPs for providing telestroke services are becoming more relevant.

TELESTROKE AND APPS

APPs are an integral part of the healthcare system in the United States. This is also true regarding telestroke care. APPs are involved in every clinical aspect of telestroke.

- At stroke hospitals, APPs often perform the physical exam on the patient while collaborating with the vascular neurologist via telestroke. APPs are involved in decision-making to provide acute stroke therapy to eligible patients.
- APPs are often the first point of contact for patients who are transferred to the hub hospital.
- APPs specialized in neurovascular disorders provide follow-up consultation using telestroke networks in both inpatient and outpatient settings.

References

Lazarus, G., Permana, A. P., Nugroho, S. W., Audrey, J., Wijaya, D. N., & Widyahening, I. S. (2020). Telestroke strategies to enhance acute stroke management in rural settings: A systematic review and meta-analysis. *Brain and Behavior, 10*(10), e01787. https://doi.org/10.1002/brb3.1787

Nelson, R. E., Saltzman, G. M., Skalabrin, E. J., Demaerschalk, B. M., & Majersik, J. J. (2011). The cost-effectiveness of telestroke in the treatment of acute ischemic stroke. *Neurology, 77*(17), 1590–1598. https://doi.org/10.1212/WNL.0b013e318234332d

Tumma, A., Berzou, S., Jaques, K., Shah, D., Smith, A. C., & Thomas, E. E. (2022). Considerations for the implementation of a telestroke network: A systematic review. *Journal of Stroke and Cerebrovascular Diseases: The Official Journal of National Stroke Association*, *31*(1), 106171. https://doi.org/10.1016/j.jstrokecerebrovasdis.2021.106171

Zachrison, K. S., Cash, R. E., Adeoye, O., Boggs, K. M., Schwamm, L. H., Mehrotra, A., & Camargo, C. A. (2022). Estimated population access to acute stroke and telestroke centers in the US, 2019. *JAMA Network Open*, *5*(2), e2145824. https://doi.org/10.1001/jamanetworkopen.2021.45824

13

End-of-Life Care

Diane McLaughlin

Advances in stroke care and efforts to prevent early withdrawal in potentially survivable conditions have made the need for palliative consultation somewhat confusing. The phrase "self-fulfilling prophecy" is when a patient is given a grave prognosis on arrival and then, subsequently, aggressive measures are not taken and the patient dies. However, end-of-life decisions must consider the patient's prestroke quality of life and values. The goal of this chapter is to give some useful information about talking to families about end-of-life care in stroke.

PROGNOSTICATION

- Prior to making a prognostic statement, clinicians should understand what is important to the patient (ability to communicate, ability to walk, acceptable level of disability) to help frame the subsequent discussion.
- There is inherent uncertainty regarding some aspects of neurological prognosis. Some structural damage has clearly identifiable subsequent outcomes, but other findings may make it hard for the provider to give clear expectations of potential recovery. Explicit disclosure of prognostic uncertainty to the family may be reasonable.
- Certain stroke syndromes have known risk for early mortality or disability, including basilar artery occlusion or malignancy middle cerebral artery infarction.
- Withdrawal bias exists, meaning that care is withdrawn prior to when the "true prognosis" is ascertained. This is more common in intracerebral hemorrhage (ICH) than other stroke types.
- It is reasonable to request a second opinion when prognostic uncertainty exists to aid the family in decision-making.

FAST FACTS

Many stroke scales have associated mortality estimations. These alone should not dictate goals of care discussions or aggressiveness of treatment.

INTUBATION/TRACHEOSTOMY

- Intubation may be needed to facilitate treatment (thrombectomy, surgery) or to protect the patient's airway. For someone with large frontal lobe infarction or hemorrhage, it is reasonable to discuss the potential need for tracheostomy down the line.

FAST FACTS

Intubation of a patient in acute respiratory failure should NOT be delayed in patients that have unclear trajectory or goals of care to facilitate these conversations. Aggressive care should be maintained to preserve all options for the patient.

- Early weaning from ventilator and extubation are desirable, as delays in extubation increase morbidity and mortality.
- In patients with structural lesions affecting the ability to protect the airway, early tracheostomy may aid in liberating patients from mechanical ventilation and facilitate earlier transfer to inpatient rehabilitation.
- In patients that elect to forgo intubation and become Do-Not-Intubate (DNI), families should be encouraged to also consider Do-Not-Resuscitate (DNR) as cardiac arrest and acute respiratory failure often coexist.

SURGICAL INTERVENTION

- In patients with hemispheric stroke (large ICH, acute ischemic stroke [AIS] with malignant edema), decompressive craniectomy can reduce mortality and increase chance of survival, albeit with moderate disability (Darsie & Moheet, 2017). Expected disability should be discussed prior to decision-making.

FAST FACTS

Current available research demonstrates improvement in quality-adjusted life years for patients aged 60 years or younger undergoing decompressive hemicraniectomy for hemispheric strokes with large areas of brain edema. In patients older than this, the benefit of this procedure is unknown.

- Current guidelines recommend that patients with large cerebellar strokes (ICH or AIS) that have neurological deterioration, brainstem

compression, or obstructive hydrocephalus typically benefit from emergent decompression (Holloway et al., 2014).
- Even in poor-grade subarachnoid hemorrhage, initial aggressive treatment is recommended, including mechanical ventilation, ventriculostomy, and aneurysmal securement if the patient can be stabilized.

PALLIATIVE CARE

- Refers to optimization of quality of life, rather than quantity by prevention and treatment of suffering
- Patient- and family-centered care
- Can be offered while still actively attempting to cure or treat underlying problems (e.g., palliative care can be offered while continuing mechanical ventilation)
- Focuses on peace, dignity, and comfort in both life and death
- Can be delivered in a multitude of care settings, including critical care, the emergency department, general hospital floors, acute rehabilitation units, nursing homes, home, or hospice

HOSPICE

- Hospice is typically reserved for patients with an anticipated life expectancy of less than 6 months.
- Inpatient hospice may be reserved for patients with an even shorter life expectancy.
- Therapies focused on curing the underlying terminal condition are discontinued.

ESTABLISHING GOALS OF CARE

Conversations regarding end-of-life and patient desires can be difficult for many providers. These should not be considered "one and done" conversations, but serial discussions to reestablish understanding of the current situation, treatment plan, and alignment with patient values.

- Start conversations with what the family's current knowledge of the situation is.
- Clarify the patient's status with what is known and not known.
  - "We know your loved one had a stroke. We know the brain area that controls language has been affected, and they will not be able to communicate with us. We do not know if they will require artificial means for nutrition."
- Find out what is important to the patient.
  - "For some patients, the act of eating and speaking are crucially important to their happiness. Other patients are happy just to be in the presence of their loved ones."
  - This helps to start the framework for decision-making.
- Give clear choices and expected consequences.
  - "Feeding is vital for human life. If a feeding tube is not placed, your loved one will die."

- Give timeframes for decision-making, but be flexible.
  - "We typically like to make decisions regarding tracheostomy when the patient has been on the ventilator 10 to 14 days; however, if you don't think your loved one would want tracheostomy, it may make sense to continue past that point if we think we can improve the odds of extubation being successful."
  - The phrase "time-limited trial" can sometimes be useful to families when watching for improvement.
- Goals of care can change as the patient's condition changes—sometimes for the better, sometimes for the worse.
- End the conversation with a clear definition of what has been determined to avoid ambiguity.
  - "We know, if your loved one's heart stops, we will focus on keeping them comfortable and not performing chest compressions or shocks."
  - "If your loved one needs a breathing tube, we know that you are okay with us doing this, even if temporarily, while you consider if they would or would not want tracheostomy."

COMMUNICATION TECHNIQUES

- Arrange family meetings that allow uninterrupted time for dialogue between the healthcare team and the family.
- Physical techniques, such as maintaining eye contact, maintaining an open posture, and sitting at the same level as families improve communication.
- Allow families a chance to be active participants and express their feelings, fears, and questions. Listen attentively and repeat to ensure understanding.
- Avoid using the phrase "I'm sorry" as it can be misinterpreted. Empathizing with the phrase "I wish" can be a good replacement.
  - "I wish we had better treatments to help your loved one."
  - "I wish you weren't having to make these decisions."
- Use the word *dying*. Families often need to hear the actual term to understand when a situation is grave.
  - "I called this meeting because I believe your loved one is dying."

REMOVAL OF LIFE SUPPORT

- Ensure hospital policies have been followed prior to initiating removal of support.
  - Organ procurement organizations often require notification prior to removal of life support.
  - Some institutions require two physicians to agree that a condition is terminal.
  - Verify if a DNR order is in place.
- Explicitly describe what will take place to the family and give them the option to be present for the physical removal of support devices.
  - Explain what medications are being ordered/administered and why.
  - Explain what the dying process will look like:

        - Likely poor responsiveness
        - Potential for anxiety, delirium
        - Pain-management regimen, moaning
        - Changes in respiratory patterns
            - Cheyne-stokes respirations
            - Apnea
            - "Death rattle" or terminal secretions
        - Arrhythmias
    - Give an estimation of the time-frame using inexact terms.
        - "We can never be certain, but we anticipate your loved one will pass in ..."
            - Minutes to hours
            - Hours to days
            - Days to weeks
- Medications at time of withdrawal
    - Pain
        - Morphine is typically preferred analgesic due to short half-life
            - Can be administered as continuous IV infusion, intermittent IV pushes, enteral formulation, or sublingual drops
    - Anxiety
        - Benzodiazepines, such as lorazepam (Ativan), alprazolam (Valium), or midazolam (Versed)
    - Hallucinations
        - Haloperidol (Haldol)
    - Terminal secretions
        - Scopolamine patch
        - Glycopyrrolate (Robinul)
        - Sublingual atropine
            - Ensure this is given as sublingual drop, as can cause pupils to acutely dilate if given as eye drop
    - Nausea
        - Ondansetron (Zofran)

PRONOUNCEMENT OF DEATH

- Assess for responsiveness to verbal and physical stimuli.
- Assess pupil response; fixed and dilated in death.
- Palpate pulse (carotid).
- Listen for cardiopulmonary effort.
- If on telemetry, determine asystole in two leads.

FAST FACTS

If mechanical ventilation remains in place, mechanical breaths may still be present, but without cardiac effort. Ensure no spontaneous respiratory effort.

Example of death note:

> Called for asystole on monitor. On physical examination, there is no response to verbal or physical stimuli. Pupils are fixed and dilated. No palpable pulse. Absent heart and lung sounds. (If on mechanical ventilation, state absent heart sounds, no spontaneous respirations.) Asystole verified in two leads. Time of death: Date/Time. Family notified at bedside.

References

Darsie, M. D., & Moheet, A. M. (2017). *The pocket guide to neurocritical care: A concise reference for the evaluation and management of neurologic emergencies.* Neurocritical Care Society.

Holloway, R. G., Arnold, R. M., Creutzfeldt, C. J., Lewis, E. F., Lutz, B. J., McCann, R. M., Rabinstein, A. A., Saposnik, G., Sheth, K. N., Zahuranec, D. B., Zipfel, G. J., Zorowitz, R. D., American Heart Association Stroke Council, Council on Cardiovascular and Stroke Nursing, & Council on Clinical Cardiology. (2014). Palliative and end-of-life care in stroke: A statement for healthcare professionals from the American Heart Association/American Stroke Association. *Stroke*, *45*(6), 1887–1916. https://doi.org/10.1161/STR.0000000000000015

Primary and Secondary Stroke Prevention

Jean Dougherty Luciano and Kathy J. Morrison

Primary prevention of stroke is generally focused on the management of vascular risk factors and lifestyle factors. Management of vascular risk factors, as with any medical management requires a comprehensive assessment of the individual, including comorbidities, resources, and social determinants of health. It is estimated that up to 90% of strokes are preventable with control of vascular risk factors and targeting multiple risk factors has an additive effect (Kleindorfer et al., 2021). In addition, awareness of familial tendencies such as aneurysms, arteriovenous malformations (AVMs), and sickle cell disease provides an opportunity for monitoring and primary prevention of hemorrhagic stroke. Secondary prevention strategies are dependent upon stroke etiology determination: large artery atherosclerosis (LAA), cardioembolism (CE), small-artery occlusion/lacune (SAO), stroke of other determined etiology (rare causes), and stroke of undetermined etiology (cryptogenic). Each of these subtypes has been shown to have distinct treatments important in secondary prevention. Chapter 11 contains comprehensive details of stroke etiology and treatment in the section on Trial of ORG 10172 in Acute Stroke Treatment (TOAST) criteria.

VASCULAR RISK FACTORS

Hypertension

- Primary prevention guidelines recommend lifestyle changes—weight loss, healthy low-sodium diet, and physical activity for borderline blood pressure (BP; 120–129/80 mmHg) and medication management for BP >130/80 mmHg.
- Secondary prevention guidelines recommend medication management with goal <130/80 mmHg.

- Medical regimens for stroke patients with hypertension (HTN) should consider patient comorbidities when determining appropriate drug classification.
- Thiazide diuretics, angiotensin-converting enzyme (ACE) inhibitors, or angiotensin II receptor blockers (ARBs) are appropriate options for both HTN management and secondary prevention (Level of evidence [LOE] 1A; Kleindorfer et al., 2021).
- Monitoring of response to antihypertensive regimens is essential, with particular attention to noncompliance and barriers to obtaining medications.
- Home BP monitoring is recommended as adjunctive to office monitoring. Instruction on proper use of the equipment and process is an important component as well as support for a tracking and reporting strategy for BP readings.

Smoking

- Cigarette smoking is an independent risk factor for ischemic stroke.
- Smoking is approximated to double the risk of stroke (Kleindorfer et al., 2021).
- Smoking cessation should be recognized as an addiction requiring both behavioral and pharmacological interventions.
- Despite experiencing a life-threatening vascular event such as a stroke, about one-third of all individuals who were premorbid smokers continue to smoke (van den Berg et al., 2019).
- Smoking cessation strategies, including counseling and drug therapy, should be considered. Options for medical therapies may include nicotine products, bupropion, or varenicline (LOE 1A; Kleindorfer et al., 2021).

Diabetes

- In the United States, it is reported that approximately 9% of adults have a diagnosis of diabetes (Bullard et al., 2018).
- Undiagnosed diabetes is discovered in approximately 20% of patients presenting with ischemic stroke (Kernan et al., 2005).
- HbA1c (hemoglobin A1c) is diagnostic for diabetes, representing an average of blood glucose for the preceding 6 weeks. The goal for secondary prevention of stroke is HbA1c <7% (LOE 1A; Kleindorfer et al., 2021).
- Cardioprotective effects of glucagon-like peptide-1 (GLP-1) receptor agonists in the setting of acute stroke and diabetes support the addition of a GLP-1 receptor agonist; therapy should be added to antihyperglycemics regardless of baseline HbA1c (Arnott et al., 2020).
- For primary prevention, lifestyle management, inclusive of maintenance of ideal body weight and a regular exercise routine, contributes to the control of diabetes as well as overall cardiovascular health.

Lipids

- For patients with ischemic stroke with no known coronary heart disease, no major cardiac sources of embolism, and low-density lipoprotein cholesterol

(LDL-C) >100 mg/dL, atorvastatin 80 mg daily is indicated to reduce risk of stroke recurrence according to the Stroke Prevention by Aggressive Reduction of Cholesterol Levels (SPARCL) study (LOE 1A; Kleindorfer et al., 2021).

- Individuals with atherosclerotic disease and stroke, in addition to statin therapy, should add ezetimibe, if needed, to a goal LDL-C of <70 mg/dL (LOE 1A; Kleindorfer et al., 2021).
- Proprotein convertase subtilisin/kexin type 9 (PCSK9) inhibitor therapy is indicated for high-risk individuals who, despite treatment with statin and ezetimibe, continue to have LDL-C >70 mg/dL (LOE 2aB-NR; Kleindorfer et al., 2021).
- Guidelines for the monitoring of lipids address monitoring of general population surveillance, not those with an acute event. In patients with stroke, an appropriate trajectory to monitor their response to medical therapy and lifestyle changes is to complete a lipid panel at baseline, 4 to 12 weeks after statin initiation or dose adjustment, and every 3 to 12 months thereafter (LOE 1A; Kleindorfer et al., 2021).
- Laboratory monitoring of liver functions should be done at baseline, 3 months post statin initiation, and then annually.

Atrial Fibrillation

- Atrial fibrillation (AF) is a prevalent risk factor for stroke, especially for older adults. It is a factor in both primary and secondary stroke prevention.
- Screening for AF during the index hospitalization as well as ambulatory monitoring with an external or implanted device is recommended if stroke etiology has not been determined (often referred to as cryptogenic stroke).
- Anticoagulation is recommended for treatment of AF if the patient has no contraindications.
- Anticoagulation agents may include direct oral anticoagulants (DOAC) or warfarin (goal international normalized ratio [INR] of 2.0–3.0).
- For patients with nonvalvular AF who have contraindications to extended anticoagulation, it may be reasonable to consider percutaneous closure of the left atrial appendage with the Watchman device. These patients must be able to tolerate at least 24 days of anticoagulation (Holmes et al., 2014).
- Monitoring of heart rate and rhythm at primary care provider (PCP) visits provides the opportunity to detect and treat AF before a stroke/transient ischemic attack (TIA) occurs.

Extracranial Carotid Artery Disease

- Extracranial carotid artery disease is a modifiable cause of stroke.
- Patients with severe stenosis ipsilateral to a nondisabling stroke should have an intervention to correct the stenosis (Kleindorfer et al., 2021).
- Anatomical considerations as well as concomitant medical conditions should be deliberated in the decision process between carotid endarterectomy or carotid artery stenting.
- Subsequent to intervention, medical management of atherosclerosis, including HTN management, lipid management, and antithrombotic should be considered along with other comorbidities.

- Auscultation of carotids for bruit at PCP visits provides the opportunity to detect and treat asymptomatic carotid stenosis before a stroke/TIA occurs. If stenosis is <70%, antithrombotic, statin, and lifestyle management are recommended. If stenosis is >70%, carotid endarterectomy or carotid stent is recommended.

FAST FACTS

Stroke patients with symptomatic intracranial atherosclerosis may benefit from short-term dual antiplatelet therapy—the combination of aspirin and clopidogrel—however, long-term dual therapy is not recommended for any stroke patients (Kleindorfer et al., 2021).

LIFESTYLE FACTORS

Diet

- In both primary and secondary prevention of stroke, the Mediterranean diet is highly recommended. The Mediterranean diet emphasizes fish and plant-based foods such as legumes, whole grains, vegetables, fruits, nuts and seeds, and olive oil.
- In hypertensive patients, it is reasonable to recommend that individuals reduce their sodium intake by at least 1 g/d sodium (2.5 g/d salt). Recommend the dietary approaches to stop hypertension (DASH) diet (LOE 2aB-R; Kleindorfer et al., 2021).

Activity

- Regular physical activity supports overall cardiovascular health. Primary prevention recommendation is for 40 min/d, 3 to 4 d/wk (Meschia et al., 2014).
- Post stroke activity should be customized to the tolerance of the patient, as stroke survivors are prone to adopting a sedentary lifestyle. Secondary prevention recommendation is for 10 min 4×/wk at minimum (LOE 1C-LD; Kleindorfer et al., 2021).
- Physical activity may have additional benefits of improving cognitive function and reducing depression (Billinger et al., 2014).

High BMI

- Current guidelines:
  - Overweight: Body mass index (BMI) 25 to 29 kg/m^2
  - Obese: 30 to 39 kg/m^2
  - Morbid obesity: >40 kg/m^2
- Both primary and secondary prevention involve weight reduction with goal of <25 kg/m^2

FAST FACTS

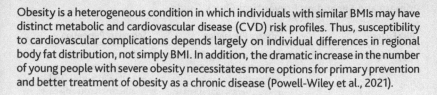

Obesity is a heterogeneous condition in which individuals with similar BMIs may have distinct metabolic and cardiovascular disease (CVD) risk profiles. Thus, susceptibility to cardiovascular complications depends largely on individual differences in regional body fat distribution, not simply BMI. In addition, the dramatic increase in the number of young people with severe obesity necessitates more options for primary prevention and better treatment of obesity as a chronic disease (Powell-Wiley et al., 2021).

Five risk factors account for 90% of ischemic and hemorrhagic strokes: HTN, poor diet, physical inactivity, smoking, and abdominal obesity (Kleindorfer et al., 2021). In Table 14.1, these five risk factors are highlighted.

TABLE 14.1

Primary and Secondary Prevention Quick Guide

Risk Factor	Primary Prevention	Secondary Prevention
HTN a. Borderline: 120–129/80 mmHg b. Stage 1: 130–139/80–89 mmHg c. Stage 2: >140/90 mmHg	a. Lifestyle changes: Weight loss, healthy, low-sodium diet, physical activity b. Medication, lifestyle changes; target <130/80 mmHg c. Same as b	Medications: thiazide diuretic, ACE I, ARB, in addition to lifestyle changes with goal of office follow-up BP <130/80 mmHg
Smoking	Behavioral modification and/or medication for cessation	Same as primary prevention
Physical Inactivity	Moderate-to-vigorous intensity physical activity at least 40 min/d 3 to 4 d/wk	Moderate physical activity at least 10 min/d, 4 d/wk or vigorous physical activity at least 20 min/d, twice a week; addition of exercise class and counseling may be beneficial
Unhealthy Diet	DASH-style diet, or Mediterranean diet supplemented with nuts; reduced sodium	Mediterranean diet; reduced sodium
High BMI ▪ Overweight: BMI 25–29 kg/m^2 ▪ Obese: BMI 30–39 kg/m^2 ▪ Morbid Obesity: >40 kg/m^2	Weight reduction with goal of BMI <25 kg/m^2	Referral to behavioral lifestyle-modification program for weight reduction with goal of BMI <25 kg/m^2
Diabetes	Glucose-lowering medications to maintain Hgb A_1C <7.0%; tight BP control; statin therapy	Glucose-lowering medications to maintain HgbA_1C <7; nutritional therapy; diabetes self-management education

(*continued*)

TABLE 14.1 (*continued*)

Primary and Secondary Prevention Quick Guide

Risk Factor	Primary Prevention	Secondary Prevention
Hyperlipidemia	■ LDL <160 mg/dL: statin; lifestyle changes ■ Family history of cardiovascular disease and LDL <160 mg/dL: statin; lifestyle changes	■ LDL <100 mg/dL: statin; lifestyle changes ■ LDL <70 mg/dL and atherosclerotic disease: statin plus ezetimibe
AF a. Valvular AF with CHA_2DS_2-VASc score of ≥2 b. Nonvalvular AF with CHA_2DS_2-VASc score of ≥ 2 c. Nonvalvular AF with CHA_2DS_2-VASc score of 0 or 1	a. Warfarin with a target INR of 2.0 to 3.0 b. Oral anticoagulants warfarin (INR, 2.0–3.0) ■ Dabigatran ■ Apixaban ■ Rivaroxaban ■ Closure of the left atrial appendage if intolerant of anticoagulants c. No antithrombotics	a. Warfarin with a target INR of 3.0 b. Oral anticoagulants warfarin (INR, 2.0–3.0) ■ Dabigatran ■ Apixaban ■ Rivaroxaban ■ Closure of the left atrial appendage if intolerant of anticoagulants
Carotid Artery Stenosis *Asymptomatic:* a. <70% stenosis b. >70% stenosis *Symptomatic:* Extracranial: a. 50% stenosis ipsilateral to stroke Intracranial: b. >50% to 69% stenosis ipsilateral to stroke c. ≥70% stenosis ipsilateral to stroke	a. Aspirin and statin; lifestyle changes b. Carotid endarterectomy or stent	a. Carotid endarterectomy within 2 weeks; antiplatelet, lipid-lowering and HTN therapies b. Aspirin 325 mg/d c. Aspirin 325 mg/d; SBP <140 mmHg; statin; moderate physical activity

ACE, angiotensin-converting enzyme; AF, atrial fibrillation; ARB, angiotensin II receptor blocker; BMI, body mass index; BP, blood pressure; DASH, dietary approaches to stop hypertension; HTN, hypertension; INR, international normalized ratio; LDL, low-density lipoprotein; SBP, systolic blood pressure.

Source: From Morrison, K. (2023). *Stroke nursing certification review*. Springer Publishing Company.

ADDITIONAL MODIFIABLE RISK FACTORS

Sleep-Disordered Breathing

- Loud snoring and sleep apnea are associated with increased carotid atherosclerosis, cardiomyopathy, AF, and HTN.
- Recommendation is to maintain healthy weight to reduce risk of snoring and to treat sleep apnea.

Hormone Therapy

- Postmenopausal hormone therapy with estrogen and/or progestin increases stroke risk.
- High-dose estrogen patches increase stroke risk at any age.
- Recommendation is to use alternate therapies to control menopausal symptoms and to avoid high-dose patches for birth control.

Migraine With Aura

- Young women with migraines who also smoke and take oral contraception have a nine-fold increased risk of stroke.
- Recommendation is to avoid triggers and take medication to control migraines; do not smoke; and use an alternate form of contraception.

Alcohol Consumption

- Heavy alcohol use (more than 21 drinks per week) is associated with HTN, hypercoagulability, reduced cerebral blood flow, and AF.
- Recommendation is two drinks or less per day for men and one drink or less per day for women.

Drug Abuse

- Cocaine, amphetamines, and heroin are linked to HTN, cerebral vasospasm, vasculitis, infectious endocarditis, increased blood viscosity, and intracranial hemorrhage (ICH).
- Recommendation is to avoid use of these drugs.

Hypercoagulability

- Hypercoagulability increases the likelihood of clot formation.
- Recommendation is to screen stroke patients under age 50 with no other etiology identified; if present, treatment with anticoagulation may be initiated.

Inflammation

- Chronic conditions, such as rheumatoid arthritis and lupus, have been associated with initiation, growth, and destabilization of atherosclerotic plaque.
- Recommendation is to avoid triggers and take medications to control these chronic conditions.

FAST FACTS

It is important to improve stroke awareness and provide education to PCPs and gynecologists regarding women at younger ages because of (a) women having an increased risk of stroke with age; (b) the risks of stroke associated with pregnancy, gestational HTN, and hormonal contraception; and (c) the onset of stroke risk factors such as obesity, HTN, and diabetes at younger ages.

NONMODIFIABLE RISK FACTORS

There are five risk factors for stroke that are not able to be modified with lifestyle changes, medication, or interventions. Individuals with one or more of the following should be managed closely with their modifiable risk factors.

Age

- Risk doubles with each decade after age 55.
- Recent studies have shown that the incidence of stroke is rising among young adults.
- A 44% increase in hospitalizations for stroke has occurred in those aged 24 to 44 years, attributed to the rise in type 2 diabetes, hypercholesterolemia, and obesity in children and young adults.
- A 29% decrease was seen in those aged 65 to 84 years, attributed to better control of risk factors like HTN, cholesterol, and diabetes (Béjot et al., 2016).

Gender

- Annually, ~55,000 more females than males have a stroke.
- Incidence rates are substantially lower in females than males in younger and middle-aged groups, but that changes after age 55 when the incidence rates in females are approximately equal to or even higher than those in males (Virani et al., 2021).

Low Birth Weight

- Risk is more than double for adults who were born with a birth weight below 2,500 g (5 lb, 8 oz).

Race/Ethnicity

- Black people have the highest incidence of stroke in the United States and a higher death rate from stroke than any other racial group.
- Over two-thirds of Black populations have at least one risk factor for stroke, with high BP being most common.
- Black and Hispanic females ≥70 years of age had higher risk of stroke compared with White females; this increased risk was not present with older Black or Hispanic males compared with White males.
- Hispanic, non-Hispanic White, Pacific Islander, and Native American populations have similar incidence of stroke. Fifty percent of Hispanic men and 40% of Hispanic women have heart disease, HTN, and diabetes.
- Stroke incidence in Hispanic people is expected to rise by 29% (Virani et al., 2021).

Genetics

- Coagulopathies and intracranial aneurysms have been shown to have familial tendencies: Marfan syndrome, sickle cell disease, and Fabry disease are associated with increased stroke risk.

- Parental ischemic stroke by the age of 65 years was associated with a threefold increase in ischemic stroke risk in offspring (Benjamin et al., 2018).
- Variants in the HDAC9 gene, as well as chromosome 9p21, have been associated with large-artery stroke.
- A variant on chromosome 16q24.2 has been associated with small vessel stroke. Variants on chromosomes 205, PMF1, and SLC25A44 and the apolipoprotein E (APOE) gene have been linked to ICH.

References

Arnott, C., Li, Q., Kang, A., Neuen, B. L., Bompoint, S., Lam, C. S. P., Rodgers, A., Mahaffey, K. W., Cannon, C. P., Perkovic, V., Jardine, M. J., & Neal, B. (2020). Sodium-glucose cotransporter 2 inhibition for the prevention of cardiovascular events in patients with type 2 diabetes mellitus: A systematic review and meta-analysis. *Journal of the American Heart Association, 9*, e014908. https://doi.org/10.1161/JAHA.119.014908

Béjot, Y., Delpont, B., & Giroud, M. (2016). Rising stroke incidence in young adults: More epidemiological evidence, more questions to be answered. *Journal of the American Heart Association, 5*(5), e003661. https://doi.org/10.1161/JAHA.116.003661

Benjamin, E. J., Virani, S. S., Callaway, C. W., Chamberlain, A. M., Chang, A. R., Cheng, S., Chiuve, S. E., Cushman, M., Delling, F. N., Deo, R., de Ferranti, S. D., Ferguson, J. F., Fornage, M., Gillespie, C., Isasi, C. R., Jiménez, M. C., Jordan, L. C., Judd, S. E., Lackland, D., … Muntner, P. (2018). Heart disease and stroke statistics—2018 update: A report from the American Heart Association. *Circulation, 137*(12), e67–e492. https://doi.org/10.1161/CIR.0000000000000558

Billinger, S. A., Arena, R., Bernhardt, J., Eng, J. J., Franklin, B. A., Johnson, C. M., MacKay-Lyons, M., Macko, R. F., Mead, G. E., Roth, E. J., Shaughnessy, M., Tang, A., On behalf of the American Heart Association Stroke Council, Council on Cardiovascular and Stroke Nursing, Council on Lifestyle and Cardiometabolic Health, Council on Epidemiology and Prevention, & Council on Clinical Cardiology. (2014). Physical activity and exercise recommendations for stroke survivors: A statement for healthcare professionals from the American Heart Association/American Stroke Association. *Stroke, 45*, 2532–2553. https://doi.org/10.1161/STR.0000000000000022

Bullard, K. M., Cowie, C. C., Lessem, S. E., Saydah, S. H., Menke, A., Geiss, L. S., Orchard, T. J., Rolka, D. B., & Imperatore, G. (2018). Prevalence of diagnosed diabetes in adults by diabetes type—United States 2016. *Morbidity and Mortality Weekly Report, 67*, 359–361. https://doi.org/10.15585/mmwr.mm6712a2

Holmes, Jr. D. R., Kar, S., Price, M. J., Whisenant, B., Sievert, H., Doshi, S. K., Huber, K., & Reddy, V. Y. (2014). Prospective randomized evaluation of the watchman left atrial appendage closure device in patients with atrial fibrillation versus longterm warfarin therapy: The PREVAIL trial. *Journal of the American College of Cardiology, 64*, 1–12. https://doi.org/10.1016/j.jacc.2014.04.029

Kernan, W. N., Viscoli, C. M., Inzucchi, S. E., Brass, L. M., Bravata, D. M., Shulman, G. I., & McVeety, J. C. (2005). Prevalence of abnormal glucose tolerance following a transient ischemic attack or ischemic stroke. *Archives of Internal Medicine, 165*, 227–233. https://doi.org/10.1001/archinte.165.2.227

Kleindorfer, D. O., Towfighi, A., Chaturvedi, S., Cockroft, K. M., Gutierrez, J., Lombardi-Hill, D., Kamel, H., Kernan, W. N., Kittner, S. J., Leira, E. C., Lennon, O., Meschia, J. F., Nguyen, T. N., Pollak, P. M., Santangeli, P., Sharrief, A. Z., Smith, Jr. S. C., Turan, T. N., & Williams, L. S. (2021). 2021 guideline for the prevention of stroke in patients with stroke and transient ischemic attack: A guideline from the American

Heart Association/American Stroke Association. *Stroke*, *52*(7), e364–e467. https://doi.org/10.1161/STR.0000000000000375

Meschia, J. F., Bushnell, C., Boden-Albala, B., Braun, L. T., Bravata, D. M., Chaturvedi, S., Creager, M. A., Eckel, R. H., Elkind, M. S., Fornage, M., Goldstein, L. B., Greenberg, S. M., Horvath, S. E., Iadecola, C., Jauch, E. C., Moore, W. S., Wilson, J. A., On behalf of the American Heart Association Stroke Council, Council on Cardiovascular and Stroke Nursing, Council on Clinical Cardiology, Council on Functional Genomics and Translational Biology, & Council on Hypertension. (2014). Guidelines for the primary prevention of stroke: A statement for healthcare professionals from the American Heart Association/American Stroke Association. *Stroke*, *45*, 3754–3832. https://doi.org/10.1161/STR.0000000000000046

Powell-Wiley, T., Poirier, P., Burke, L., Després, J., Gordon-Larsen, P., Lavie, C., Lear, S. A., Ndumele, C. E., Neeland, I. J., Sanders, P., St-Onge, M., On behalf of the American Heart Association Council on Lifestyle and Cardiometabolic Health, Council on Cardiovascular and Stroke Nursing, Council on Clinical Cardiology, Council on Epidemiology and Prevention, & Stroke Council. (2021). Obesity and cardiovascular disease: A scientific statement from the American Heart Association. *Circulation*, *143*, e984–e1010. https://doi.org/10.1161/CIR.0000000000000973

van den Berg, M. J., van der Graaf, Y., Deckers, J. W., de Kanter, W., Algra, A., Kappelle, L. J., de Borst, G. J., Cramer, M. M., Visseren, F. L. J., & SMART Study Group. (2019). Smoking cessation and risk of recurrent cardiovascular events and mortality after a first manifestation of arterial disease. *American Heart Journal*, *213*, 112–122. https://doi.org/10.1016/j.ahj.2019.03.019

Virani, S. S., Alonso, A., Aparicio, H. J., Benjamin, E. J., Bittencourt, M. S., Callaway, C. W., Carson, A. P., Chamberlain, A. M., Cheng, S., Delling, F. N., Elkind, M. S. V., Evenson, K. R., Ferguson, J. F., Gupta, D. K., Khan, S. S., Kissela, B. M., Knutson, K. L., Lee, C. D., Lewis, T. T., … Tsao, C. W. (2021). Heart disease and stroke statistics—2021 update: A report from the American Heart Association. *Circulation*, *143*(8), e254–e743. https://doi.org/10.1161/CIR.0000000000000950

15

Provider and Staff Education and Competency

Kaylie Yost, Catherine Mielke, and Karen Pratt

Education, training, and competency are not intended to be interchangeable terms. Competency is supported by the delivery of education and training.

- **Education** ***is defined by The Joint Commission as the process of receiving systematic instruction resulting in the acquisition of theoretical knowledge.***
- **Training** ***focuses on gaining specific, often manually performed, technical skills***
- **Competency** ***incorporates knowledge, technical skill and ability which develops after the receipt of and participation in education and training.***

EDUCATION

- Initial education
    - Several programs exist for purchase that are kept up to date with evidence-based practice.
        - Apex Innovations offers comprehensive guideline-based coursework that encompasses stroke management for clinicians of all levels. Free National Institutes of Health Stroke Scale (NIHSS) coursework is available through the company.
        - Organizations can develop original educational content. The up-to-date performance measures, evidence-based practice, and American Heart Association Stroke Guidelines should be utilized for development of learning objectives.
- Ongoing education
    - It is advisable to ensure that the ongoing education content is selected to meet the needs of the staff who care for the patients.
    - Certain topics of education (i.e., NIHSS, tissue plasminogen activator [tPA], TNKase, cerebrovascular disease, etc.) should be delivered annually, while others may be more beneficial to be placed in a biannual rotation of topics.

    - If the organization chooses to seek certification, it is imperative that staff complete the identified hours of education on stroke-related topics (see Table 15.1).
- Just-in-time education
  - Near-miss and sentinel events can signal the need for reinforcement of education.
  - New procedures/protocols that are implemented quickly can be benefitted by providing at-the-elbow support and education for the initial users.

TRAINING

- Training for specific skills can be best accomplished by offering staff the opportunity to complete the skill in the most realistic environment possible. Doing so offers the learners the best opportunity to be able to retain the skill.
- Consider the use of standardized patients in simulation centers and mock events.
- Debriefing after training sessions can prove effective to highlight additional opportunities for training or education prior to the evaluation of competency (Table 15.2).

TABLE 15.1

Staff Education Requirements for Primary and Comprehensive Stroke Program Certification

Staff Role	Annual Education Required (Hours)
Core stroke team members	8 (must be stroke education)[a]
ED RNs	2 (must be cerebrovascular disease)[a]
Non-nursing ED staff Physician assistants, EKG technicians, respiratory care technicians, imaging staff, laboratory staff, and so forth as identified by the organization	2 (must be cerebrovascular disease)[a]
Nurses (other than ED) caring for comprehensive stroke patients as identified by the organization. Examples may include, but are not limited to, nurses providing stroke care in the stroke unit, ICU that contains the dedicated neurointensive care beds for complex stroke patients, endovascular catheterization laboratory, patient care units, a rehabilitation unit, and so forth.	8 (must be stroke education)[a]

[a]Applicable Standards—Delivering or Facilitating Clinical Care: DSDF.1 EP 7.
Source: From The Joint Commission. (2022). *Advanced DSC—Comprehensive stroke manual.* https://store.jcrinc.com/2023-certification-standards-books/2023-stroke-certification-standards-manual-pdf-manual-/

TABLE 15.2

Educational Responsibilities

Designated Education Coordinator Responsibilities	Staff Responsibilities
■ Monitor competency program ■ Monitor staff progress ■ Facilitate competency assessment ■ Coordinate with subject matter experts to develop competencies that are in alignment with evidence-based practice and organizational policies and procedures ■ Evaluate competency program	■ Participate in brainstorming for competency development ■ Complete identified initial and annual competencies ■ Evaluate competency program

FAST FACTS

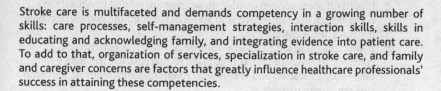

Stroke care is multifaceted and demands competency in a growing number of skills: care processes, self-management strategies, interaction skills, skills in educating and acknowledging family, and integrating evidence into patient care. To add to that, organization of services, specialization in stroke care, and family and caregiver concerns are factors that greatly influence healthcare professionals' success in attaining these competencies.

COMPETENCY

- Identification of competencies
  - Competency identification follows the following progression:
    - Competency identification is an evolving process that occurs throughout the year (Table 15.3). Consider the following when brainstorming: high risk, new, changes, and/or problematic (Wright, 2005).
      - Prioritize feedback from brainstorming sessions
      - Complete learning needs assessment

TABLE 15.3

Annual Competency Timeline

Quarter 1	Quarter 2	Quarter 3	Quarter 4
Make final decisions for the current calendar year competency topics based on the brainstorming completed in quarter 4 of the previous year	Development of competency topics and answer guides	Evaluation of competency assessment	Completion of current year competency Begin the brainstorming process for the next calendar year competency assessments

- When identifying competencies, it is important to consider and include the following:
  - Staff input (current bedside staff, clinicians, team leaders/charge nurses)
  - Quality metrics and data
  - Performance measures
  - Regulatory requirements for specialty certifications
  - National Patient Safety Goals published by The Joint Commission
  - Environmental scanning
  - Root cause analysis
  - Hospital initiatives
- Initial and ongoing competency
  - Competencies that are deemed high risk are beneficial to be completed upon initial hire and annually to maintain proficiency.
  - Selected annual competencies should be meaningful to the staff who must complete them.
  - Identify if there are gaps and if those gaps are related to education, competency, accountability, and so forth through the completion of a learning needs assessment.
  - If your organization has a low volume of high-risk patients (i.e., complex stroke patients), it is advised to increase the frequency of delivering education and training to maintain proficiency of staff who care for stroke patients.
- Evaluation of competency
  - There are several ways to evaluate competency. Those mentioned in Table 15.4 have proven effective for staff who care for patients who have been diagnosed with or are being evaluated for a stroke.

TABLE 15.4

Competency Evaluation Techniques

Method	Domain	Explanation
Mock events	Assess response in daily work or practice	Provides opportunity for debrief, self-reflection, individual performance, identification of additional needs
Return demonstration	Technical/ psychomotor skills	Measured by a skilled observer
Case studies	Critical thinking skills	Case study must match the competency being measured
Test/exam	Measure of retention of cognitive information	Is there retention of the information being measured for the specified competency? Does not demonstrate performance or psychomotor skills
Evidence of daily work	Technical domain	Job skill proficiency demonstrated on a daily basis

- Staff should be provided with resources and tools necessary to prepare them to exhibit competency. At the time when competency is evaluated, there should not be delivery of coaching or education.
- If the staff member fails to successfully demonstrate a specific competency, a remediation plan should be developed and discussed. Once remediation has been completed, they can attempt to have their competency evaluated for accuracy.
- Simulations/return demonstrations
  - Return demonstration for use of equipment and utilization of standardized patients where available to practice NIHSS are both recommended

CERTIFICATION REQUIREMENTS

Organizations can choose to apply for stroke program certification. The institution should pick which certifying body best meets the needs of their organization.

- Performance measures are useful in guiding the selection of topics for education and training of staff (see Chapter 2 for performance measures).
- Always ensure that the current requirements of the certifying body are being followed. Updates occur and it is the organization's responsibility to ensure criteria are met.

FAST FACTS

Education for staff who work in specialty areas (ED, ICU, stroke unit) should include documentation of education in NIHSS, dysphagia screening, and tPA administration per the organization's requirements (The Joint Commission, 2022).

ADDITIONAL INFORMATION

- Workgroups and committees dedicated to management of stroke patients have proven effective at ensuring patients are receiving efficient, appropriate care within the guidelines outlined by certification centers such as The Joint Commission and Det Norske Veritas (DNV).
  - Successful facilities utilize a stroke coordinator and a stroke clinical practice committee to review collected data and identify opportunities for improvement within the organization.
- Specialty certifications are encouraged for those providing care to stroke patients:
  - Emergency Neurological Life Support—Neuro Critical Care Society offers this certification to a variety of healthcare professional roles
  - Advanced Cardiac Life Support—American Heart Association
  - Certified Neuroscience Registered Nurse—American Board of Neuroscience Nursing
  - Stroke Certified Registered Nurse—American Board of Neuroscience Nursing

References

The Joint Commission. (2022). *Quick guide to primary stroke center certification*. Joint Commission. https://www.jointcommission.org/-/media/tjc/documents/accred-and-cert/certification/certification-by-setting/stroke/psc-quick-guide---psc-4-9-digital.pdf

Wright, D. K. (2005). *The ultimate guide to competency assessment in health care*. Creative Health Care Management.

16

Quality Metrics, Data Use, and Guidelines

Claranne Mathiesen

Since the Institute of Medicine (IOM) published To Err is Human: Building a Safer Health System *in 1999, hospitals have placed an increasing emphasis on evidence-based care and quality initiatives. This has created a much-needed momentum to improve the quality of healthcare. Several frameworks have helped to apply this to the care of patients with stroke and transient ischemic attack. Quality activities are designed to close the gap between evidence (what is recommended in the guidelines) and practice (evaluated with data collected on quality of care provided; Kilkenny & Bravata, 2021). Using a cycle in which data is collected and analyzed to address a question and then fed back to a healthcare team drives the quality improvement process. This aligns with the plan, do, study, and act model. Another approach to assessing quality is using the Donabedian model (Figure 16.1) looking at structure, processes, and outcomes (Donabedian, 1988).*

As a busy advanced practice provider (APP), it is important to have a handle on performance improvement activities and utilize data to drive clinical decision-making. Some questions to help drive use of data include:

- *What is this data measuring? Familiarity with the data and clarity of what is being measured will give credibility in driving improvements.*
- *How big of a sample is this representing? It is h to get excited on only one or two cases that do not meet the metric goal, often called "fallouts."*
- *Is this a mean or a median being reported? Mean is the average of a group of values, while median is the value sitting at the midpoint of a frequency distribution of a group of values. The two values might be similar, depending on the data, but extreme outliers will skew the mean much more than the median.*
- *Who is responsible for this metric? Some of the stroke core measures are timed by provider documentation occurring at specific points in care (Hint: Is your APP documentation telling the story you want?).*

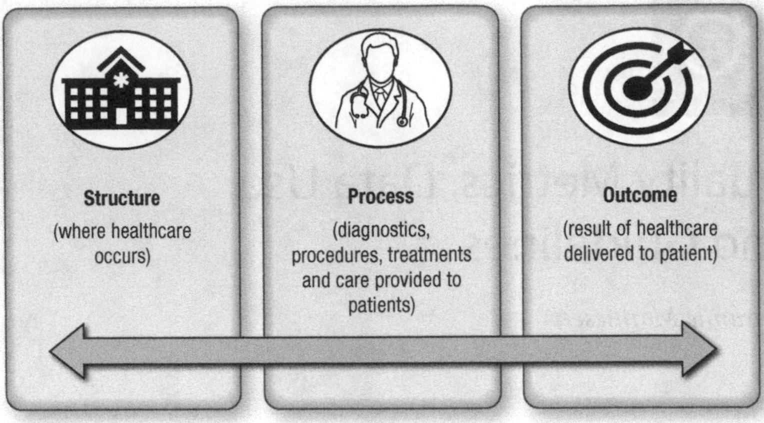

Figure 16.1 Adaptation of Donabedian healthcare quality model.

Source: Adapted from Donabedian, A. (1988). The quality of care. *JAMA*, 1743–1748. https://doi.org/10.1001/jama.260.12.1743

QUALITY METRICS

There are many different quality measures applied to the stroke patient population. Keeping track can sometimes be challenging, but more than likely if you look at the role you play in delivering stroke patient care, you will have some targets to achieve. Additionally, healthcare systems also place an increasing emphasis on certain quality indicators such as length of stay, readmissions, and stroke mortality, and it is not uncommon to have hospital-wide goals (for example, decreasing length of stay or reducing preventable readmissions).

COMMON DATA MEASURES

- Core measures: standardized, defined measures that are collected related to a process or outcome (i.e., standardized stroke core measure set).
- Brain attack measures: process measures developed by Brain Attack Coalition to measure timeliness of care in the ED (i.e., door to provider, door to CT, door to drug).
- Quality achievement measures: additional quality measures that are recognized as contributing to quality care (i.e., American Heart Association [AHA] Get With The Guidelines [GWTG] stroke quality measures).
- Outcome measures: measure an outcome of care (i.e., length of stay, readmission, stroke order set usage).

ROLE OF THE APP AS PART OF THE QUALITY TEAM

1. APPs play a key role in driving care for stroke patients. This often includes using order sets, reviewing diagnostic results, modifying stroke risk

factors, providing patient education on treatments for stroke, and helping to evaluate stroke care systems.
2. As part of the interdisciplinary team, APPs often collaborate to ensure evidence-based care delivery occurs and may identify opportunities across the system for change.
3. APPs additionally help to communicate across the continuum and assist with making smooth transitions to different healthcare settings.
4. Hospital APPs are critical to ensuring that the plan of care is clearly documented so that appropriate follow-up occurs in the outpatient setting.
5. Some APPs are key members of the stroke leadership team and may contribute to creating and executing the stroke program performance improvement plan.
6. Often APPs partner with the stroke coordinator and stroke medical director to assist in ongoing performance improvement activities.
7. APPs in the primary care office assist with primary and secondary prevention. They also help with ensuring patients have been connected to outpatient resources for ongoing recovery poststroke.
8. APPs often are part of the team in specialty care offices ensuring workup is complete and new risk factors are treated. As many stroke patients follow in multiple areas, the APP assists with communication of plan of care.
9. APPs across all settings have grown in their role supporting delivery of stroke care especially as navigators emerge with making sure that care transitions are seamless, communication between services are clear, and patient/caregiver education is ongoing (Chilakamarri et al., 2021).

DATA USE

Since 2000 when Brain Attack Coalition published its recommendations for the establishment of stroke centers, many hospitals have taken a closer look at how they provide stroke care. Over the last two decades, different levels of certified stroke centers have evolved. These continue to be recognized as we further develop interactions within our stroke systems of care model. Data has also been an important part of how hospitals share key information on internal performance as well as been used by external agencies to rate how hospitals may perform (Amini et al., 2020). The use of a stroke registry provides clear benefits in standardizing reporting, optimizing data collection tools, and allowing benchmarking against others.

FAST FACTS

Benchmarking refers to the use of either internal or external best practices to drive performance improvement efforts. For example, the use of another organization's reported reduction of stroke readmission after incorporating APPs in their stroke clinic is a form of benchmarking. Sharing this best practice and result, along with a plan to replicate it, will have greater success with the hospital administration (Figures 16.2, 16.3, 16.4, and 16.5).

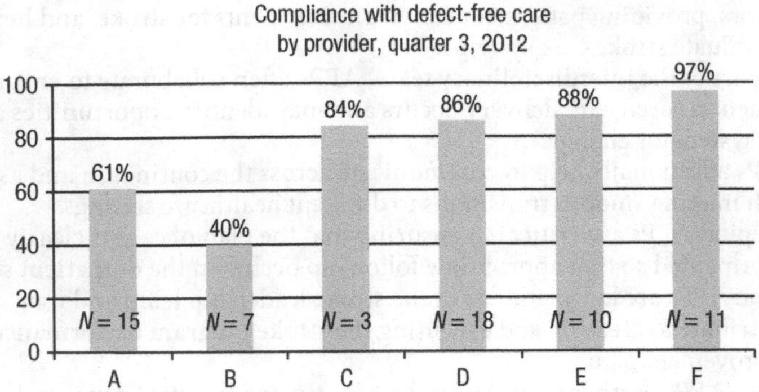

Figure 16.2 Report card for providers: Blinded format stimulates curiosity as to who is the most compliant.

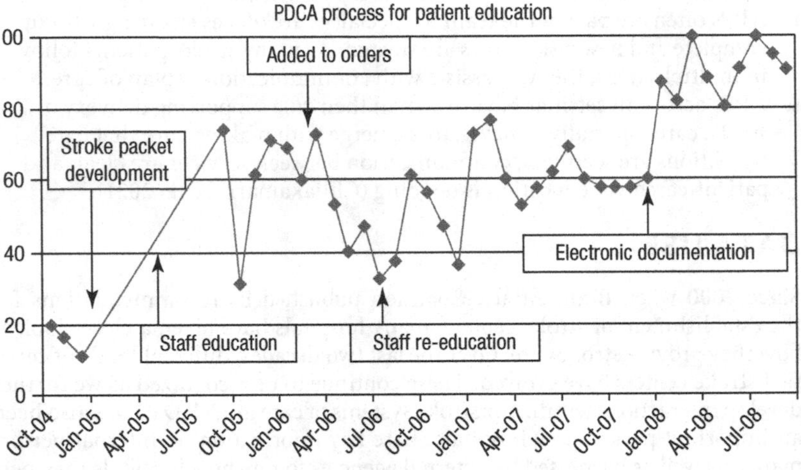

Figure 16.3 Compliance over time, with key actions to show impact.

Source: From Morrison, K. (2018). *Fast facts for stroke care nursing* (2nd ed.). Springer Publishing Company.

DATABASES

Internal Data Sources

Internal data sources provide organizations with the abilities to identify stroke patients and track them during a hospital stay.

- Stroke log: This is usually maintained by the stroke coordinator to provide key data points for process and outcomes of stroke patients (essential for Stroke Center certification).

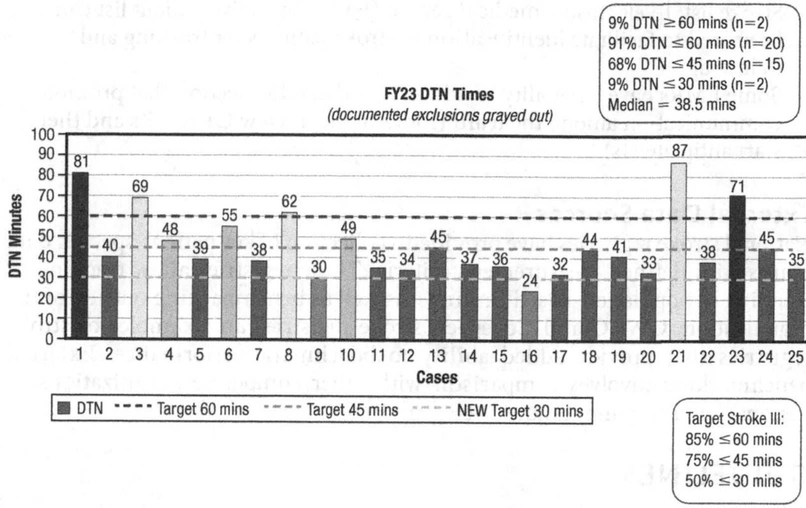

Figure 16.4 Door-to-needle times example.

Note: An example of door-to-needle (DTN) times at one organization; this format facilitates comparison of all thrombolytic cases in a given timeframe. Includes outpatients only, exludes tPA given prehospital, data from Stroke Alert/tPA log.

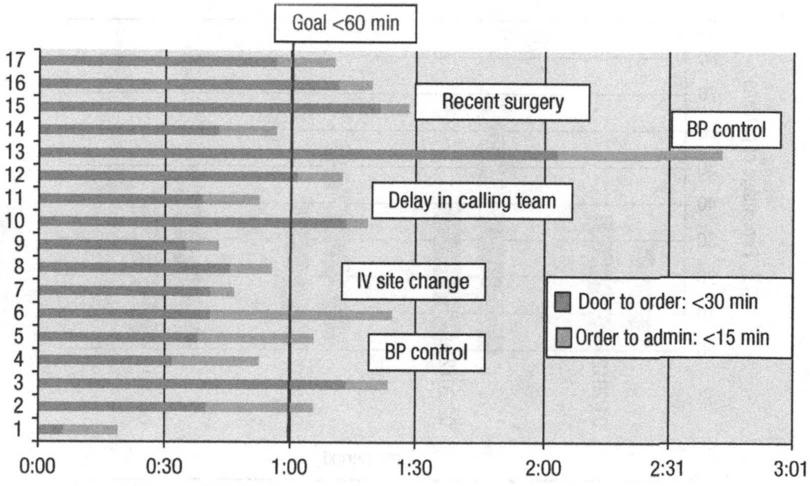

Figure 16.5 Door-to-needle times graph.

Note: Format provides details that illustrate where in the treatment process delays occurred. *Source:* From Morrison, K. (2018). *Fast facts for stroke care nursing* (2nd ed.). Springer Publishing Company.

- Stroke list: In electronic medical record (EMR), an active patient list can be shared to facilitate identification of stroke patients for tracking and follow-up.
- Some EMRs have the ability to add a "to do" handoff section that promotes communication among the team (for example, review CT results and then start antiplatelets).

External Data Sources

National stroke registries have provided a collection of key patient-specific data points with defined measurement criteria. These registries allow tracking or trending of population-based findings, as well as benchmarking outside of the organization. GWTG and Coverdell stroke registries are examples of stroke registries that provide added ability to benchmark performance. External benchmarking involves comparison with other competing organizations or national/international standards (Figure 16.6).

GUIDELINES

Clinical practice guidelines are systematically developed statements to assist practitioner and patient decisions about appropriate healthcare for specific clinical circumstances (Field & Lohr, 1990).

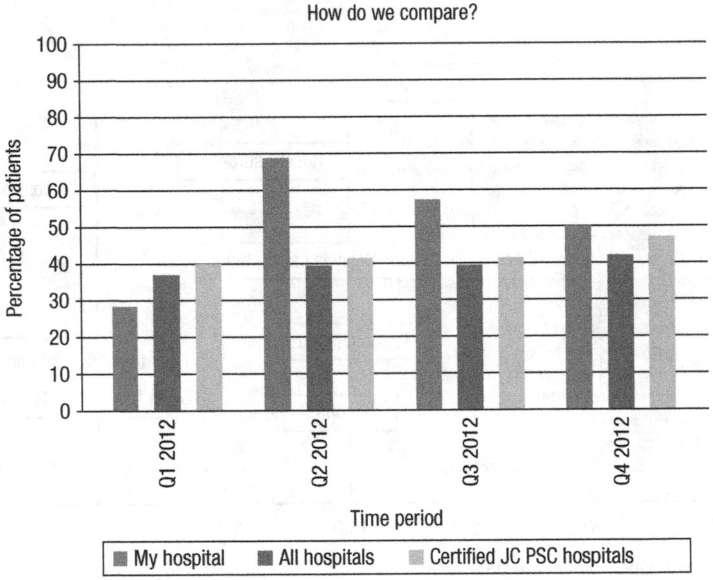

Figure 16.6 Door-to-needle times.

Note: Comparison with other certified centers to facilitate competitive spirit.
Source: From Morrison, K. (2018). *Fast facts for stroke care nursing* (2nd ed.). Springer Publishing Company.

- Evidence summary providing best practices on acute stroke care
- Externally validated by subject matter experts
- Internally reviewed and adopted by clinicians at your local practice site and integrated into care pathways, care bundles, and stroke order sets; require periodic review for accuracy and currency and are often evaluated as part of certification and accreditation visits
- APPs have an important role as guideline users and often drive adoption of new evidence at the bedside.

Sample Stroke Guidelines

Below is a list of sample stroke guidelines. This is not meant to be an exhaustive list. Additionally, stroke guidelines are always being updated, so check frequently.

- Neurocritical Care Society: www.neurocriticalcare.org/resources/guidelines
- American Heart Association: https://professional.heart.org/en/guidelines-and-statements/guidelines-and-statements-search
- Society of NeuroInterventional Surgery: www.snisonline.org/standards/
- Society for Vascular Surgery: https://vascular.org/vascular-specialists/practice-and-quality/clinical-guidelines/clinical-guidelines-and-reporting

Strategies for When Guidelines Change or Are Updated

When guidelines are changing or updating, they are distributed to a group of impacted stakeholders to evaluate what is new or different from current practices. Changes should be made available to the stroke team, nursing units, key physicians and APPs, and practice council and key leadership groups.

To ensure that guidelines remain evidence-based, revisions need to include internal documents (policies, pathways, and procedures manuals), as well as order set changes. Information can be disseminated to journal clubs, through team meetings, via tip sheets and job aides (i.e., post on unit, badge buddies, and pocket cards), electronically (orders, best practice advisory pop ups), and through e-learning modules.

FAST FACTS

The APP who is familiar with the stroke guidelines and facilitates other healthcare team members' familiarity will find greater engagement in providing high-quality evidence-based care.

References

Amini, M., van Leeuwen, N., Eijkenaar, F., Mulder, M., Schonewille, W., Lycklama à Nijeholt, G., Hinsenveld, W. H., Goldhoorn, R. J. B., van Doormaal, P. J., Jenniskens, S., Hazelzet, J., Dippel, D. W. J., Roozenbeek, B., Hester, F., & Lingsma on behalf of the MR CLEAN Registry Investigators. (2020). Improving quality of stroke care through benchmarking center performance: Why focusing on outcomes is not enough. *BMC Health Services Research*, *20*(1), 1–10. https://doi.org/10.1186/s12913-020-05841-y

Chilakamarri, P., Finn, E. B., Sather, J., Sheth, K. N., Matouk, C., Parwani, V., Ulrich, A., Davis, M., Pham, L., Chaudhry, S. I., & Venkatesh, A. K. (2021). Failure mode and effect analysis: Engineering safer neurocritical care transitions. *Neurocritical Care*, *35*, 232–240. https://doi.org/10.1007/s12028-020-01160-6

Donabedian, A. (1988). The quality of care. *JAMA*, *260*(12), 1743–1748. https://doi.org/10.1001/jama.260.12.1743

Field, M. J., & Lohr, K. (1990). Clinical practice guidelines: Directions for a new program. *Committee to Advise Public Health Service on Clinical Practice Guidelines.* https://doi.org/10.1007/978/-1-4419-1005-9_1113

Kilkenny, M. F., & Bravata, D. M. (2021). Quality improvement. *Stroke*, *52*(5), 1866–1870. https://doi.org/10.1161/STROKEAHA.121.033451

17

Stroke Research and the Advanced Practice Provider

Emily Rogers

Advances in stroke research extend throughout the entire continuum of care including prevention, acute intervention, and recovery. Over the last half century, considerable advances have greatly shaped the incidence and outcomes associated with stroke. This includes the development of active treatment which contrasts greatly from prior nihilistic and passive approaches (Anderson, 2021). APRNs and other advanced practice providers (APPs) possess foundational knowledge of research methodology that allows for evaluation and implementation of relevant data into practice. Maintaining awareness of current and forthcoming research is essential for the APP to advocate for patients as well as population outcomes.

WHERE TO BEGIN IN DISCOVERING RESEARCH

Professional Organizations

- Provide clinical practice guidelines (CPG) comprised of systematic reviews of data as well as alerts for new updates in care
- Annual conferences provide networking and dissemination opportunities for APPs to engage in collaboration of new scientific research (Goolsby & DuBois, 2017).
- Multiple options for stroke-focused APPs including:
  - American Stroke Association
  - American Association of Neuroscience Nurses
  - American Association of Neurology
  - Neurocritical Care Society
- The National Institute of Neurologic Disorders and Stroke (NINDS) created the National Institutes of Health (NIH) StrokeNet as a network for healthcare professionals to access and collaborate for the benefit of stroke research (Broderick et al., 2016; Frasure & Spilker, 2018).

- Open platform for small and large clinical trials
  - Includes all stage II and III multisite (>5 sites) trials with NIH funding
  - Provides access to current trial information in a concise format organized by prevention, acute intervention, and recovery and rehabilitation trials
  - Includes additional details for each trial, such as summary, design, outcomes, and status or enrollment updates
  - Network includes 27 regional centers with approximately 500 hospitals in the United States; also has international collaborative sites
  - Includes educational offerings such as webinars and recorded presentations

RECENT UPDATES IN STROKE

Stroke Systems

National certification of stroke centers results in improved care and outcomes; tiered levels of stroke centers include:

- Acute stroke ready hospitals
- Primary stroke centers
- Thrombectomy-capable stroke centers
- Comprehensive stroke centers

Additionally, high-volume centers have been associated with improved outcomes in subarachnoid hemorrhage (SAH; Rush et al., 2017). Further validation of finding was found when adjusted for severity of SAH.

Mobile Stroke Units

Another area of research includes mobile stroke units. Mobile stroke units typically consist of ambulance response which includes en route CT capability and thrombolysis.

- B_PROUD 2.0 trial demonstrated decreased time to thrombolysis and endovascular intervention with use of mobile stroke unit (Bender et al., 2022)
- BEST-MSU trial subsequently demonstrated improved functional outcomes at 90 days

Ischemic Stroke

Traditional therapy focuses on prompt recognition, appropriate imaging, and timely thrombolysis or thrombectomy if indicated. Recognition and grading of stroke symptoms is often reliant upon scales such as the NIH Stroke Scale (NIHSS).

- NIHSS has preferential assessment for anterior circulation stroke and can underestimate severity of posterior circulation stroke.
- ASPOS: Adams Scale of Posterior Stroke
  - Seven-item scored assessment (reactivity, eyes, pharynx, strength, balance, ataxia, and sensory)
  - Validity and reliability demonstrated on prospective, observational study
- Artificial intelligence applications in stroke imaging remain a discussion point in patient selection and require further research (Pilato et al., 2021; Wardlaw et al., 2022).
- Time limited candidacy criteria for thrombolysis and mechanical thrombectomy are continuously under evaluation.

THROMBOLYSIS

For thrombolysis, the benefit versus risk of alteplase therapy outside of 4.5 hours from last known well time has been highly reviewed. Systematic review and meta-analysis of prior interventional studies include EXTEND, ECASS4-EXTEND, and EPITHET to evaluate thrombolysis from 4.5 to 9 hours (Table 17.1; Ringleb et al., 2019).

- Improved functional outcomes with alteplase compared to placebo therapy, although higher rate of symptomatic intracranial hemorrhage (ICH)

TABLE 17.1

Thrombolysis

Study	Objective	Pitfalls	Bottom Line
NINDS (NINDS, 1995)	Evaluating tPA with window of 3 hours **Primary Outcomes:** 1. NIHSS improvement of 4 points, resolution within 24 hours 2. Barthel index, Modified Rankin Scale, Glasgow outcome scale, NIHSS at 3 months	Placebo group had more severe stroke (NIHSS >20), fewer mild stroke (NIHSS 0–5)	IV tPA is beneficial in 3 hour time frame
ECASS III (Hacke et al., 2008)	Evaluating tPA with window of 3–4.5 hours **Primary Outcome:** Modified Rankin Scale at 90 days	More narrow selection criteria than NINDS, excluded: Large strokes (NIHSS >25), prior anticoagulation, prior stroke, DM, age >80	IV tPA is beneficial in 3–4.5 hour time frame Favorable mRS at 90 days
TOAST (1998)	**Primary Outcome:** Barthel Index, Glasgow Outcome Score measured at 7 days and 3 months		No benefit of heparin over aspirin for acute strokes (<24 hours)
EXTEND (Ma et al., 2019)	Evaluating tPA with window of 4.5–9 hours with salvageable tissue on CT perfusion or perfusion-diffusion MR imaging **Primary Outcomes:** 1. Modified Rankin Scale at 90 days 2. Percentages of reperfusion at 24 hours	Increased symptomatic ICH in tPA group	IV tPA is beneficial in 4.5–9 hour time frame

(*continued*)

TABLE 17.1 (*continued*)

Thrombolysis

Study	Objective	Pitfalls	Bottom Line
ECASS IV EXTEND (Amiri et al., 2016)	Evaluating tPA with window of 4.5–9 hours with salvageable tissue on MR imaging **Primary Outcomes:** 1. Modified Rankin Scale at 90 days 2. Percentages of reperfusion at 24 hours	Increased symptomatic ICH in tPA group	No benefit
EPITHET (Davis et al., 2008)	Evaluating tPA with window of 3–6 hours with perfusion mismatch on MR imaging **Primary Outcomes:** 1. Modified Rankin Scale at 90 days 2. Percentages of reperfusion at 24 hours		No difference in benefit with age >80; tPA improves reperfusion in patients with penumbra

DM, diabetes mellitus; ECASS, European Cooperative Acute Stroke Study; EPITHET, Echoplanar Imaging Thrombolytic Evaluation Trial; EXTEND, extending the time for thrombolysis in emergency neurological deficits; ICH, intracranial hemorrhage; mRS, magnetic resonance spectroscopy; NIHSS, The National Institutes of Health Stroke Scale; NINDS, National Institute of Neurological Disorders and Stroke; TOAST, Trial of ORG 10172 in Acute Stroke Treatment; tPA, tissue plasminogen activator.

Tenecteplase

Additionally, tenecteplase has been evaluated for efficacy compared to alteplase therapy. Prospective, observational cohort comparisons have demonstrated improved door to needle time, door-in-door-out time, and reduced cost (Table 17.2; Katsanos et al., 2021; Warach et al., 2022).

Mechanical Thrombectomy

For mechanical thrombectomy, the studies listed in Table 17.3 established a new standard of perfusion guided selection with extension of candidacy for mechanical thrombectomy to 24 hours after last known well.

Specific approaches to mechanical thrombectomy have also been evaluated.

- Comparative approaches include direct aspiration or stent retriever for evaluation of efficacy.
  - Findings were suggestive of comparable outcomes although variables proved challenging to control, including operator preference and anatomical differences.

TABLE 17.2

Tenecteplase

Study	Objective	Pitfalls	Bottom Line
NOR-TEST I (Rønning et al., 2019) NOR-TEST II (Kvistad et al., 2022)	Evaluating tenecteplase (0.4 mg/kg dose) versus alteplase with 3–4.5 hours **Primary Outcome:** 1. Modified Rankin Scale at 90 days	NOR-TEST II was terminated early due to increased rate of symptomatic ICH	Tenecteplase was as effective as alteplase in low NIHSS although increased rates of hemorrhage found with worse outcomes in subsequent study of mild to moderate NIHSS
ATTEST (Huang et al., 2015) ATTEST II trial currently ongoing	Evaluating tenecteplase (0.25 mg/kg) dose versus alteplase within 4.5 hours **Primary Outcome:** Penumbra salvaged	Single center trial	Tenecteplase

ATTEST, alteplase-tenecteplase for thrombolysis after ischemic stroke; ICH, intracranial hemorrhage; NIHSS, The National Institutes of Health Stroke Scale; NOR TEST, Norwegian Tenecteplase Stroke Trial.

TABLE 17.3

Mechanical Thrombectomy

Study	Objective	Pitfalls	Bottom Line
DEFUSE III (Albers et al., 2018)	Evaluating thrombectomy within 6–16 hours after last known well time Primary outcome: 1. Modified Rankin Scale at 90 days	Specialized imaging and intervention limit generalizability	MT 6–16 hours after symptom onset improves outcomes
DAWN (Nogueira et al., 2018)	Evaluating thrombectomy with Trevo device 6–24 hours after last known well time Primary outcome: 1. Modified Rankin Scale at 90 days	Industry sponsored with single device Patients with smaller area of infarct (<10 mL) but higher enrollment NIHSS	MT 6–24 hours after symptom onset improves outcomes

(continued)

TABLE 17.3 (*continued*)

Mechanical Thrombectomy

Study	Objective	Pitfalls	Bottom Line
AURORA (Jovin et al., 2022) Analysis of pooled pata from randomized studies of thrombectomy more than 6 hours after last known well time	Primary outcome: 1. Modified Rankin Scale at 90 days		In patients with evidence of reversible ischemia, MT 6–24 hours after symptom onset improves outcomes
EXTEND IA TNK (Campbell et al., 2018)	Evaluating TNK versus tPA prior to thrombectomy Primary outcomes: 1. Revascularization of greater than 50% of blood flow of involved territory or absence of thrombus 2. Modified Rankin Scale at 90 days	Open label due to dosing differences Noninferiority study	TNK noninferior to TPA with improved functional outcome in TNK group Data had trend towards higher reperfusion in TNK group No significant increase in symptomatic ICH

AURORA, A study to evaluate the use of rosuvastatin in subjects on regular hemodialysis; DAWN, Diffusion-Weighted Imaging or CTP Assessment With Clinical Mismatch in the Triage of Wake-Up and Late Presenting Strokes Undergoing Neurointervention With Trevo; EXTEND, extending the time for thrombolysis in emergency neurological deficits; ICH, intracranial hemorrhage; MT, medical transcription; NIHSS, The National Institutes of Health Stroke Scale; TNK, tenecteplase; tPA, tissue plasminogen activator.

HEMORRHAGIC STROKE

ICH Management

The management of ICH continues to provide opportunities for improved outcomes. Recent clinical updates include severity scoring.

- ICH score is widely utilized for severity grading in ICH.
- Mortality prediction derived from the traditional ICH score has been shown to overestimate mortality in severe ICH (≥4) when maximal medical therapy is utilized.
- Max-ICH score includes more specific criteria derived from age, NIHSS, ICH volume and location, and use of anticoagulation. Max-ICH score was subsequently validated in a multicenter trial which demonstrated improved prognostication of functional outcome after ICH when compared to the ICH score (Sembill et al., 2021).

Hypertension Management

The management of hypertension remains an area of great discussion and ongoing evaluation. INTERACT2 (Second Intensive Blood Pressure Reduction in Acute Cerebral Hemorrhage Trial) and Antihypertensive Treatment of Acute Cerebral Hemorrhage II (ATACH-2) are recognized for early standards of blood pressure (BP) control in ICH (Anderson et al., 2013; Qureshi et al., 2016).

- Multiple limitations to the findings from these studies include variation from blood pressure targets within study groups (Moullaali et al., 2019).
- Secondary analysis of the data has also revealed that more rapid reduction in BP and strict control was associated with neurologic deterioration as well as cardiac adverse events and renal-related adverse events (Leasure et al., 2019).
- Guidelines have been updated to recommend (Gusler et al., 2022):
  - Initiation of treatment with avoidance of variability in systolic blood pressure
  - Presentation with:
    - Mild-to-moderate severity ICH (goal range of 130–150 mmHg may be reasonable)
    - Large or severe ICH: safety and efficacy of acute blood pressure reduction is not well established
    - Acute lowering of systolic blood pressure to <130 mmHg is potentially harmful
- Superiority of surgical evacuation of hematoma in ICH has also been challenging to demonstrate in large trials.
  - MISTIE III: minimally invasive surgery plus rt-PA for ICH evacuation
    - Open label, blinded endpoint trial which failed to demonstrate superiority to medical treatment
  - ENRICH: early minimally invasive removal of intracerebral hemorrhage
    - Industry sponsored study for the evaluation of neuralgia-inducing cavitational osteonecrosis (NICO) BrainPath and NICO myriad systems in minimally invasive evacuation of hematoma
    - May result in change in surgical management of ICH
    - Trial is complete although results are not available, but expected by the time of publication of this book
- Primary endpoints for research in SAH include endovascular intervention as well as rebleeding, vasospasm, delayed cerebral edema
  - Medical management also requires ongoing evaluation for efficacy as new knowledge and therapies are developed.

STROKE RECOVERY

- Tele-rehab is an emerging option for patients and has shown promising results in early, small sample studies (Dodakian et al., 2017).
  - This strategy assists with issues of access, such as cost and compliance issues with rehab after stroke.
    - Effective use of home-based system was demonstrated and associated with increased motor status improvement.
    - Computer literacy was not associated with variance of gains.

CURRENT AND FORTHCOMING LARGE TRIALS

- Prevention:
  - This classification encompasses primary as well as secondary prevention for stroke.
  - Significant points in this area include antiplatelet therapy, anticoagulation, and other medication regimens associated with potential benefit.
- Ischemic stroke: Prevention strategies undergoing evaluation include the reduction of vascular risk for populations such as intracranial atherostenosis and extracranial atherosclerotic disease.
  - CAPTIVA: comparison of anticoagulation and antiplatelet for intracranial vascular atherostenosis
    - The purpose of this study is to evaluate the efficacy and safety of low dose rivaroxaban or ticagrelor versus the current standard of care (clopidogrel) in the management of major intracranial artery atherostenosis with prior asymptomatic infarct.
    - Population/Enrollment: age 30 to 80, prior asymptomatic infarct attributed to 70% to 99% stenosis of major intracranial artery (middle cerebral artery, intracranial carotid, intracranial vertebral, and basilar)
      - Target enrollment: 1,683 participants
    - Multicenter randomized, double-blind, two-staged, Phase 3, 3-arm trial
      - Intensive medical treatment with:
        - Aspirin and ticagrelor therapy
        - Aspirin and rivaroxaban therapy
        - Aspirin and clopidogrel therapy (standard)
      - Primary outcome: evaluation of superiority in the novel treatment groups to standard management
      - Safety outcomes: intracranial or extracranial major hemorrhage
      - Additional exploratory aim will evaluate CYP2C19 loss-of-function carrier status benefit between arms
  - CREST-2: the carotid revascularization and medical management for asymptomatic carotid stenosis study
    - The purpose of this study is to evaluate intensive modern medical therapy to surgical intervention (including carotid endarterectomy and carotid stenting).
    - Population/Enrollment: 35 or greater years of age, 70% or greater carotid stenosis, asymptomatic (including stroke or transient ischemic attack [TIA])
      - Target enrollment: 2,480 participants
    - Multicenter, randomized, and observer-blind endpoint clinical trials
      - Intensive medical management alone versus intensive medical management with one of the following:
        - Carotid stenting
        - Carotid endarterectomy
      - Primary outcome: stroke and death within 4 years

- CREST-H: carotid revascularization and medical management for asymptomatic carotid stenosis trial-hemodynamics
  - Evaluating the subset of CREST-2 patients with mild cognitive impairment to determine if revascularization influences cognition
- Evaluation of silent embolic risk also has provided opportunities for ongoing research.
  - ARCADIA: atrial cardiopathy and antithrombotic drugs in prevention after cryptogenic stroke
    - The purpose of this study is to explore the benefit of apixaban in atrial cardiopathy (in the absence of atrial fibrillation or flutter) with prior cryptogenic stroke.
      - Atrial cardiopathy is defined as one of the following:
        - P-wave terminal force > 5,000 μV × ms in ECG lead V[1]
        - Serum NT-proBNP >250 pg/mL
        - Left atrial diameter index ≥3 cm/m² on echocardiogram
    - Population/Enrollment: 45 or greater years of age, modified Rankin Scale score <4, embolic stroke of undetermined source, evidence of atrial cardiopathy
      - Target enrollment: 1,100 participants
    - Multicenter, randomized, double-blind, active control, Phase 3 clinical trial
      - Medical management with aspirin (standard)
      - Medical management with apixaban
      - Primary outcome: recurrent stroke within 4 years
      - Safety outcomes: symptomatic intracranial or major extracranial hemorrhage
  - ARCADIA: cognition and silent infarcts (CSI)
    - Ancillary ARCADIA trial to assess for incidence of silent infarction and associated cognitive change between study arms
- Prevention of recurrent stroke in prior ICH: Studies have previously shown oral anticoagulation benefit to patients with atrial fibrillation following ICH, measured by significant reduction in thromboembolic events; however, the data has been largely observational and randomized control trials are lacking.
  - ASPIRE: anticoagulation for stroke prevention and recovery after ICH
    - The purpose of this study is to evaluate the safety and efficacy of apixaban or aspirin therapy in prevention of thromboembolic events after recent ICH
    - Population/Enrollment: 18 or greater years of age, nonvalvular AF (CHA2DS2-VASc score ≥2), single prior ICH with 14 to 120 days of entry
      - Target enrollment: 700 participants
    - Multicenter, randomized, double-blind, and Phase 3 clinical trial
      - Apixaban versus aspirin therapy
      - Primary outcome: evaluate superiority of apixaban therapy to aspirin therapy for prevention of stroke or all cause death
      - Secondary outcomes: modified Rankin Scale as well as safety and efficacy by measure of major hemorrhage, thromboembolic events, cognition and quality of life

- As with anticoagulation, use of HMG-CoA reductase inhibitors (statins) in patients with ICH is controversial; prior studies have found potential protective effect of hyperlipidemia in ICH as well as increased risk of ICH with intensive therapy (Shoamanesh & Selim, 2022).
  - SATURN: statin use in intracerebral hemorrhage patient
    - The purpose of this study is to evaluate the association between continuation of statin therapy and recurrent ICH in patients with spontaneous lobar ICH while on statin therapy.
    - Population/Enrollment: 50 years or greater age, spontaneous lobar ICH onset with 7 days of enrollment, on statin therapy at time of ICH onset
      - Target enrollment: 1,456 participants
    - Multicenter, randomized, prospective, Phase 3 clinical trial, pragmatic, open-label, and blinded endpoint
      - Continuation versus discontinuation of statin therapy
      - Primary outcome: recurrent ICH within 24 months
      - Secondary outcomes: major adverse cerebrovascular or cardiovascular events
- Acute intervention:
  - Multitiered management of stroke creates challenges in developing novel and effective treatments.
  - Interventions include imaging strategies, endovascular or surgical action, and supportive management throughout a diverse range of stroke mechanisms.
- Ischemic stroke: Traditional thrombolysis with tissue plasminogen activator (tPA) has been frequently challenged by new treatment options to evaluate for superiority.
  - MOST: multiarmed optimization of stroke thrombolysis
    - The purpose of this study is to evaluate the effectiveness of tPA in combination with argatroban or eptifibatide.
    - Population/Enrollment: 18 or greater years of age, received IV tPA within 3 hours of symptom onset and will receive study drug within 1 hour of IV tPA
      - Target enrollment: 1,200 participants
    - Multicenter, randomized, Phase 3, three-arm, blinded, controlled clinical trial
      - IV tPA and one of the following:
        - Placebo (standard)
        - Argatroban
        - Eptifibatide
      - Primary outcome: efficacy of novel treatment (IV tPA + argatroban or eptifibatide) over standard treatment by measure of 90-day modified Rankin Scale
      - Safety outcome: symptomatic ICH
  - RHAPSODY-2: recombinant variant of human activated protein C (3K3A-APC) in combination with tPA in acute hemispheric ischemic stroke

- The purpose of the study is to evaluate the safety and efficacy of 3K3A-APC in acute ischemic stroke requiring thrombolysis and/or mechanical thrombectomy.
- Population/Enrollment: 18 to 90 years of age, acute ischemic stroke requiring thrombolysis or mechanical thrombectomy, ability to receive study drug within 120 minutes of thrombolysis completion or mechanical thrombectomy start
    - Target enrollment: 1,040 participants
- Multicenter, randomized, double-blind, Phase 3, and two-phased clinical trial
    - Lead-in, dose-finding phase
        - Primary outcome: intracerebral hemorrhage or death proportion lower than control group
        - Trial will stop if target not achieved
    - Definitive phase
        - Primary outcome: 90-day disability based on modified Rankin Scale

- ICH: ICH has proven challenging for developing treatment strategies although medical and surgical modalities continue to emerge for evaluation.
    - FASTEST: recombinant factor VIIa (rFVIIa) for acute hemorrhagic stroke administered at earliest time trial
        - The purpose of the study is to evaluate the benefit of rFVIIa administered within 120 minutes of stroke onset over standard therapy.
        - Population/Enrollment: 18 to 80 years of age, spontaneous ICH, able to receive study drug within 120 minutes of onset
            - Target enrollment: 860 participants
        - Multicenter, randomized, Phase 3, double-blind, and control trial
            - Standard AHA guideline directed medical therapy and placebo versus rFVIIa injection
            - Primary outcome: modified Rankin Scale at 180 days
            - Secondary outcome: ICH growth
- SAH: Management points in SAH include vasospasm prevention and treatment.
    - REACT: prevention and treatment of vasospasm with clazosentan
        - The purpose of this study is to evaluate the effectiveness of clazosentan on cerebral vasospasm.
        - Population/Enrollment: 18 to 70 years of age, ruptured saccular aneurysm with securement within 72 hours of rupture
            - Target enrollment: 409 participants
        - Multicentered, randomized, double-blind clinical trial
            - Standard medical management and placebo versus clazosentan
        - Primary outcome: clinical deterioration due to delayed cerebral ischemia within 14 days of study drug administration
        - Secondary outcomes: cerebral infarction, functional status by modified Rankin Scale, Glasgow Outcome Scale extended

- Recovery and rehabilitation: Stroke is the leading cause of disability in adult patients in America which further supports the need for ongoing effort towards maximizing rehabilitation.
  - TRANSPORT 2: transcranial direct current stimulation for poststroke motor recovery—a Phase 2 study
    - The purpose of this study is to evaluate the benefit of transcranial direct current stimulation on unilateral limb weakness after acute ischemic stroke.
    - Population/Enrollment: 18 to 80 years of age, unilateral limb weakness following first unihemispheric ischemic stroke within 30 to 180 days prior to study enrollment
      - Target enrollment: 129 participants
    - Multicenter, Phase 2, 3-arm dosing selection study
      - Three dosing groups: sham, 2 mA, 4 mA
      - Combined with modified constraint-induced movement therapy
      - Primary outcome: treatment effect as measured by Fugl-Meyer upper-extremity scale
      - Secondary outcomes: functional motor activity, quality of life by measure of the stroke impact scale, sustained benefit at day 45 and day 105
  - VERIFY: validation of early prognostic data for recovery outcome after stroke for future, higher yield trials
    - The purpose of this study is to validate biomarkers for upper extremity motor outcome after acute stroke.
    - Population/Enrollment: 18 or greater years of age, enrolled within 48 to 96 hours of onset of acute stroke, motor deficits in acutely effected upper extremity
      - Target enrollment: 657 participants
    - Multicenter, biomarker validation trial
    - Primary outcome: external validation of transcranial magnetic stimulation (TMS) and MRI biomarkers in motor impairment
    - Secondary outcomes: external validation of additional prediction tool (PREP2), develop and validate multivariable prediction tools for the prediction of upper extremity function

References

Albers, G. W., Marks, M. P., Kemp, S., Christensen, S., Tsai, J. P., Ortega-Gutierrez, S., McTaggart, R. A., Torbey, M. T., Kim-Tenser, M., Leslie-Mazwi, T., Sarraj, A., Kasner, S. E., Ansari, S. A., Yeatts, S. D., Hamilton, S., Mlynash, M., Heit, J. J., Zaharchuk, G., Kim, S., … DEFUSE 3 Investigators. (2018). Thrombectomy for stroke at 6 to 16 hours with selection by perfusion imaging. *The New England Journal of Medicine, 378*(8), 708–718. https://doi.org/10.1056/NEJMoa1713973

Amiri, H., Bluhmki, E., Bendszus, M., Eschenfelder, C. C., Donnan, G. A., Leys, D., Molina, C., Ringleb, P. A., Schellinger, P. D., Schwab, S., Toni, D., Wahlgren, N., & Hacke, W. (2016). European cooperative acute stroke study-4: Extending the time for thrombolysis in emergency neurological deficits ECASS-4: ExTEND. *International Journal of Stroke: Official Journal of the International Stroke Society, 11*(2), 260–267. https://doi.org/10.1177/1747493015620805

Anderson, C. S. (2021). Progress in stroke: Marking the 30-year anniversary of cerebrovascular diseases. *Cerebrovascular Diseases (Basel, Switzerland)*, *50*(1), 2–3. https://doi.org/10.1159/000514399

Anderson, C. S., Heeley, E., Huang, Y., Wang, J., Stapf, C., Delcourt, C., Lindley, R., Robinson, T., Lavados, P., Neal, B., Hata, J., Arima, H., Parsons, M., Li, Y., Wang, J., Heritier, S., Li, Q., Woodward, M., Simes, R. J., … INTERACT2 Investigators. (2013). Rapid blood-pressure lowering in patients with acute intracerebral hemorrhage. *The New England Journal of Medicine*, *368*(25), 2355–2365. https://doi.org/10.1056/NEJMoa1214609

Bender, M. T., Mattingly, T. K., Rahmani, R., Proper, D., Burnett, W. A., Burgett, J. L., LEsperance, J., Cushman, J. T., Pilcher, W. H., Benesch, C. G., Kelly, A. G., & Bhalla, T. (2022). Mobile stroke care expedites intravenous thrombolysis and endovascular thrombectomy. *Stroke and Vascular Neurology*, *7*(3), 209–214. https://doi.org/10.1136/svn-2021-001119

Broderick, J. P., Palesch, Y. Y., Janis, L. S., & National Institutes of Health StrokeNet Investigators. (2016). The National Institutes of Health StrokeNet: A user's guide. *Stroke*, *47*(2), 301–303. https://doi.org/10.1161/STROKEAHA.115.011743

Campbell, B. C. V., Mitchell, P. J., Churilov, L., Yassi, N., Kleinig, T. J., Dowling, R. J., Yan, B., Bush, S. J., Dewey, H. M., Thijs, V., Scroop, R., Simpson, M., Brooks, M., Asadi, H., Wu, T. Y., Shah, D. G., Wijeratne, T., Ang, T., Miteff, F., … EXTEND-IA TNK Investigators. (2018). Tenecteplase versus alteplase before thrombectomy for ischemic stroke. *The New England Journal of Medicine*, *378*(17), 1573–1582. https://doi.org/10.1056/NEJMoa1716405

Davis, S. M., Donnan, G. A., Parsons, M. W., Levi, C., Butcher, K. S., Peeters, A., Barber, P. A., Bladin, C., De Silva, D. A., Byrnes, G., Chalk, J. B., Fink, J. N., Kimber, T. E., Schultz, D., Hand, P. J., Frayne, J., Hankey, G., Muir, K., Gerraty, R., … EPITHET Investigators. (2008). Effects of alteplase beyond 3 h after stroke in the Echoplanar Imaging Thrombolytic Evaluation Trial (EPITHET): A placebo-controlled randomized trial. *The Lancet. Neurology*, *7*(4), 299–309. https://doi.org/10.1016/S1474-4422(08)70044-9

Dodakian, L., McKenzie, A. L., Le, V., See, J., Pearson-Fuhrhop, K., Burke Quinlan, E., Zhou, R. J., Augsberger, R., Tran, X. A., Friedman, N., Reinkensmeyer, D. J., & Cramer, S. C. (2017). A home-based telerehabilitation program for patients with stroke. *Neurorehabilitation and Neural Repair*, *31*(10–11), 923–933. https://doi.org/10.1177/1545968317733818

Frasure, J., & Spilker, J. (2018). How nurses can partner with National Institutes of Health StrokeNet to deliver best research and care to stroke patients. *Stroke*, *49*(1), e1–e4. https://doi.org/10.1161/STROKEAHA.117.017872

Goolsby, M. J., & DuBois, J. C. (2017). Professional organization membership: Advancing the nurse practitioner role. *Journal of the American Association of Nurse Practitioners*, *29*(8), 434–440. https://doi.org/10.1002/2327-6924.12483

Gusler, M., Joseph, N., Quin, S., Ravishankar, K., Srinivas, M., Teitcher, M., Ulep, R., Bezanson, J. L., & Antman, E. M. (2022). *Clinical update; adapted from: 2022 guideline for the management of patients with spontaneous intracerebral hemorrhage: A guideline from the American Heart Association/American Stroke Association [PowerPoint slides]*. https://professional.heart.org/en/science-news

Hacke, W., Kaste, M., Bluhmki, E., Brozman, M., Dávalos, A., Guidetti, D., Larrue, V., Lees, K. R., Medeghri, Z., Machnig, T., Schneider, D., von Kummer, R., Wahlgren, N., Toni, D., & ECASS Investigators. (2008). Thrombolysis with alteplase 3 to 4.5 hours after acute ischemic stroke. *New England Journal of Medicine*, *359*(13), 1317–1329. https://doi.org/10.1056/NEJMoa0804656

Huang, X., Cheripelli, B. K., Lloyd, S. M., Kalladka, D., Moreton, F. C., Siddiqui, A., Ford, I., & Muir, K. W. (2015). Alteplase versus tenecteplase for thrombolysis after ischemic stroke (ATTEST): A phase 2, randomized, open-label, blinded endpoint study. *The Lancet Neurology, 14*(4), 368–376. https://doi.org/10.1016/S1474-4422(15)70017-7

Jovin, T. G., Nogueira, R. G., Lansberg, M. G., Demchuk, A. M., Martins, S. O., Mocco, J., Ribo, M., Jadhav, A. P., Ortega-Gutierrez, S., Hill, M. D., Lima, F. O., Haussen, D. C., Brown, S., Goyal, M., Siddiqui, A. H., Heit, J. J., Menon, B. K., Kemp, S., Budzik, R., … Albers, G. W. (2022). Thrombectomy for anterior circulation stroke beyond 6 h from time last known well (AURORA): A systematic review and individual patient data meta-analysis. *Lancet (London, England), 399*(10321), 249–258. https://doi.org/10.1016/S0140-6736(21)01341-6

Katsanos, A. H., Safouris, A., Sarraj, A., Magoufis, G., Leker, R. R., Khatri, P., Cordonnier, C., Leys, D., Shoamanesh, A., Ahmed, N., Alexandrov, A. V., & Tsivgoulis, G. (2021). Intravenous thrombolysis with tenecteplase in patients with large vessel occlusions: Systematic review and meta-analysis. *Stroke, 52*(1), 308–312. https://doi.org/10.1161/STROKEAHA.120.030220

Kvistad, C. E., Næss, H., Helleberg, B. H., Idicula, T., Hagberg, G., Nordby, L. M., Jenssen, K. N., Tobro, H., Rörholt, D. M., Kaur, K., Eltoft, A., Evensen, K., Haasz, J., Singaravel, G., Fromm, A., & Thomassen, L. (2022). Tenecteplase versus alteplase for the management of acute ischemic stroke in Norway (NOR-TEST 2, part A): A phase 3, randomized, open-label, blinded endpoint, non-inferiority trial. *The Lancet. Neurology, 21*(6), 511–519. https://doi.org/10.1016/S1474-4422(22)00124-7

Leasure, A. C., Qureshi, A. I., Murthy, S. B., Kamel, H., Goldstein, J. N., Woo, D., Ziai, W. C., Hanley, D. F., Al-Shahi Salman, R., Matouk, C. C., Sansing, L. H., Sheth, K. N., & Falcone, G. J. (2019). Association of intensive blood pressure reduction with risk of hematoma expansion in patients with deep intracerebral hemorrhage. *JAMA Neurology, 76*(8), 949–955. https://doi.org/10.1001/jamaneurol.2019.1141

Ma, H., Campbell, B. C. V., Parsons, M. W., Churilov, L., Levi, C. R., Hsu, C., Kleinig, T. J., Wijeratne, T., Curtze, S., Dewey, H. M., Miteff, F., Tsai, C. H., Lee, J. T., Phan, T. G., Mahant, N., Sun, M. C., Krause, M., Sturm, J., Grimley, R., … EXTEND Investigators. (2019). Thrombolysis guided by perfusion imaging up to 9 hours after onset of stroke. *The New England Journal of Medicine, 380*(19), 1795–1803. https://doi.org/10.1056/NEJMoa1813046

Moullaali, T. J., Wang, X., Martin, R. H., Shipes, V. B., Robinson, T. G., Chalmers, J., Suarez, J. I., Qureshi, A. I., Palesch, Y. Y., & Anderson, C. S. (2019). Blood pressure control and clinical outcomes in acute intracerebral haemorrhage: A preplanned pooled analysis of individual participant data. *The Lancet Neurology, 18*(9), 857–864. https://doi.org/10.1016/S1474-4422(19)30196-6

National Institute of Neurological Disorders and Stroke rt-PA Stroke Study Group. (1995). Tissue plasminogen activator for acute ischemic stroke. *The New England Journal of Medicine, 333*(24), 1581–1587. https://doi.org/10.1056/NEJM199512143332401

Nogueira, R. G., Jadhav, A. P., Haussen, D. C., Bonafe, A., Budzik, R. F., Bhuva, P., Yavagal, D. R., Ribo, M., Cognard, C., Hanel, R. A., Sila, C. A., Hassan, A. E., Millan, M., Levy, E. I., Mitchell, P., Chen, M., English, J. D., Shah, Q. A., Silver, F. L., … DAWN Trial Investigators. (2018). Thrombectomy 6 to 24 hours after stroke with a mismatch between deficit and infarct. *The New England Journal of Medicine, 378*(1), 11–21. https://doi.org/10.1056/NEJMoa1706442

Pilato, F., Calandrelli, R., Capone, F., Alessiani, M., Ferrante, M., Iaccarino, G., & Di Lazzaro, V. (2021). New perspectives in stroke management: Old issues and new pathways. *Brain Sciences, 11*(6), 767. https://doi.org/10.3390/brainsci11060767

The Publications Committee for the Trial of ORG 10172 in Acute Stroke Treatment (TOAST) Investigators. (1998). Low molecular weight heparinoid, ORG 10172 (danaparoid), and outcome after acute ischemic stroke: A randomized controlled trial. *JAMA, 279*(16), 1265–1272.

Qureshi, A. I., Palesch, Y. Y., Barsan, W. G., Hanley, D. F., Hsu, C. Y., Martin, R. L., Moy, C. S., Silbergleit, R., Steiner, T., Suarez, J. I., Toyoda, K., Wang, Y., Yamamoto, H., Yoon, B. W., & ATACH-2 Trial Investigators and the Neurological Emergency Treatment Trials Network. (2016). Intensive blood-pressure lowering in patients with acute cerebral hemorrhage. *The New England Journal of Medicine*, *375*(11), 1033–1043. https://doi.org/10.1056/NEJMoa1603460

Ringleb, P., Bendszus, M., Bluhmki, E., Donnan, G., Eschenfelder, C., Fatar, M., Kessler, C., Molina, C., Leys, D., Muddegowda, G., Poli, S., Schellinger, P., Schwab, S., Serena, J., Toni, D., Wahlgren, N., Hacke, W., & ECASS-4 Study Group. (2019). Extending the time window for intravenous thrombolysis in acute ischemic stroke using magnetic resonance imaging-based patient selection. *International Journal of Stroke: Official Journal of the International Stroke Society*, *14*(5), 483–490. https://doi.org/10.1177/1747493019840938

Rønning, O. M., Logallo, N., Thommessen, B., Tobro, H., Novotny, V., Kvistad, C. E., Aamodt, A. H., Næss, H., Waje-Andreassen, U., & Thomassen, L. (2019). Tenecteplase versus alteplase between 3 and 4.5 hours in Low National Institutes of Health Stroke Scale. *Stroke*, *50*(2), 498–500. https://doi.org/10.1161/STROKEAHA.118.024223

Rush, B., Romano, K., Ashkanani, M., McDermid, R. C., & Celi, L. A. (2017). Impact of hospital case-volume on subarachnoid hemorrhage outcomes: A nationwide analysis adjusting for hemorrhage severity. *Journal of Critical Care*, *37*, 240–243.

Sembill, J. A., Castello, J. P., Sprügel, M. I., Gerner, S. T., Hoelter, P., Lücking, H., Doerfler, A., Schwab, S., Huttner, H. B., Biffi, A., & Kuramatsu, J. B. (2021). Multicenter validation of the max-ICH score in intracerebral hemorrhage. *Annals of Neurology*, *89*(3), 474–484. https://doi.org/10.1002/ana.25969

Shoamanesh, A., & Selim, M. (2022). Use of lipid-lowering drugs after intracerebral hemorrhage. *Stroke*, *53*(7), 2161–2170. https://doi.org/10.1161/STROKEAHA.122.036889

Warach, S. J., Dula, A. N., Milling, T. J., Miller, S., Allen, L., Zuck, N. D., Miller, C., Jesser, C. A., Misra, L. R., Miley, J. T., Mawla, M., Ding, M. C., Bertelson, J. A., Tsui, A. Y., Jefferson, J. R., Davison, H. M., Shah, D. N., Ellington, K. T., Padrick, M. M., … Paydarfar, D. (2022). Prospective observational cohort study of tenecteplase versus alteplase in routine clinical practice. *Stroke*, *53*, 3583–3593. Advance online publication. https://doi.org/10.1161/STROKEAHA.122.038950

Wardlaw, J. M., Mair, G., von Kummer, R., Williams, M. C., Li, W., Storkey, A. J., Trucco, E., Liebeskind, D. S., Farrall, A., Bath, P. M., & White, P. (2022). Accuracy of automated computer-aided diagnosis for stroke imaging: A critical evaluation of current evidence. *Stroke*, *53*(7), 2393–2403. https://doi.org/10.1161/STROKEAHA.121.036204

GLOSSARY

Abulia: A lack of will or initiative

Agnosia: Failure to recognize stimuli when the appropriate sensory systems are functioning adequately; commonly occurs in visual, tactile, and auditory forms

Antithrombotics: Medications that prevent clot formation; two classes are anticoagulants and antiplatelet agents

Aphasia: Loss of ability to use language and to communicate thoughts verbally or in writing; receptive aphasia (inability to understand); expressive aphasia (inability to speak/write)

Ataxia: Lack of coordination or clumsiness of movement that is not the result of muscular weakness; it is caused by vestibular, cerebellar, or sensory disorders

Aura: Subjective sensation preceding a paroxysmal attack; may precede migraines or seizures and can be psychic or sensory in nature

Autoregulation: Ability of the cerebral vasculature to maintain stable blood flow despite changes in blood pressure

Bifurcation: Division of a blood vessel into two branches

Broca's area: Region in dominant right frontal lobe responsible for motor speech

Class of recommendation: Evidence and/or general agreement that a given treatment or procedure is beneficial, useful, effective; benefit versus risk; *see* Level of evidence

Clonic: Alternating contraction and relaxation of muscles

Collateral circulation: Circulation of blood established through enlargement of minor vessels and anastomosis of vessels with those of adjacent parts when a major vein or artery is functionally impaired (as by obstruction)

Comorbid conditions: Presence of one or more disorders in addition to the primary disorder; for example, a stroke patient with diabetes and hypertension—these are comorbid conditions

Contralateral: Originating in, or affecting, the opposite side of the body

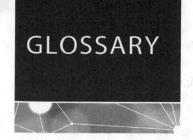

Cortical: Referring to the outer layer of the cerebrum; predominantly gray matter

Decerebrate: Posture characterized by a rigid—possibly arched—spine, rigidly extended arms and legs, and plantar flexion; indicative of a brain-stem lesion

Decorticate: Posture characterized by a rigid spine, inwardly flexed arms, extended and internally rotated legs, and plantar flexion; indicative of a brain-stem lesion

Delirium: Mental confusion and excitement characterized by disorientation for time and place, usually with illusions and hallucinations; possible causes are fever, shock, exhaustion, anxiety, or drug overdose

Dementia: An acquired, generalized, and often progressive impairment of cognitive function that affects the content, but not the level, of consciousness; may indicate pathology affecting the cerebral cortex, its subcortical connections, or both

Diffusion: Movement of molecules from a region of higher concentration to a region of lower concentration

Diplopia: Double vision; may indicate pathology involving the cranial nerves, eyeballs, cerebellum, cerebrum, or meninges

Dissection: Separation of the layers of an arterial or venous wall resulting in reduced lumen and possibly complete occlusion

Dysphagia: Difficulty swallowing or inability to swallow

Dysphasia: Impaired ability to communicate with verbal or written language; seldom used in clinical care, as aphasia has come to be used to represent not only the inability to communicate, but also the impaired ability to communicate; dysphasia is often confused with dysphagia

Euthermia: Condition of having normal body temperature; synonym is normothermia

Fissure: Deep cleft or groove between segments of the cerebral cortex; larger than a sulcus

Graphesthesia: Ability to recognize symbols when they're traced on the skin

Gray matter: Largest portion of the brain; neuronal cell bodies and glial cells in the cortex and deep nuclei process information originating in the sensory organs or in other gray matter regions

Gyrus (plural is gyri): Prominent convolutions on the surface of the cerebral hemispheres

Half-life: Time it takes for the amount of a drug's active substance in your body to reduce by half

Hemianopia: Loss of half of the visual field; homonymous hemianopia means that both right visual fields, or both left visual fields are lost

Hemicraniectomy: surgical removal of part of the skull to relieve increased intracranial pressure

Hemiparesis: Weakness affecting only one side of the body; may indicate an intracranial structural lesion

Hemiplegia: Paralysis affecting only one side of the body; may indicate pathology of upper motor neurons

Hemorrhagic transformation: Also called hemorrhagic conversion; that is, leakage of blood from vessels in the ischemic stroke bed; the presence of blood "transforms" an ischemic stroke into a hemorrhagic stroke on imaging, but improved imaging makes it possible to differentiate a primary hemorrhage from an ischemic stroke with hemorrhagic transformation

Hyperreflexia: Abnormally intense response to a stimulus; may indicate a lesion of the upper motor neurons and suggests lack of cortical control over the reflex

Hypoperfusion: Inadequate blood flow to a region of the brain

Ictal: Pertaining to or caused by a sudden attack such as acute epilepsy

Infarction: Irreversible damage or death of tissue

Inion: Point at the external occipital protuberance of the skull

Intima: Innermost lining of an artery or vein

Intrathecal: Introduction of substance into the subarachnoid space of the brain or spinal cord; certain drugs are given this way to avoid the blood–brain barrier

Ipsilateral: Originating in or affecting the same side of the body

Ischemia: Insufficient blood flow to meet metabolic demand; if not corrected, leads to hypoxia and infarction

Lenticulostriate arteries: A collection of small perforating arteries arising from the anterior part of the circle of Willis and supplying the basal ganglia

Level of evidence: Strength of the evidence supporting the recommendation; *see* Class of recommendation

Meta-analysis: Statistical analysis of the data from independent primary studies focused on the same question

Myelin: White fatty material that encloses the axons of myelinated nerve fibers; acts as an insulator, increasing the speed of transmission of nerve signals

Myoclonic: Twitching or clonic spasm of a muscle or group of muscles

Nerve palsy: Neurological defect caused by dysfunction of the nerve that controls that part of the body; for example, third cranial nerve palsy is manifested by limited eye movements and ptosis

Normothermia: Normal body temperature; synonym is euthermia

Nystagmus: Involuntary, rhythmic, oscillating motions of the eyes

Parenchyma: Functional tissue of an organ, distinguished from connective and supporting tissue

Peduncles: The structures connecting the cerebellum to the brain stem and the cerebrum

Penetrating arteries: Small, nonbranching end arteries which arise directly from larger arteries

Perfusion: Passage of fluid through the circulatory system

Pharmacokinetics: Characteristic interactions of a drug and the body in terms of its absorption, distribution, metabolism, and excretion

Plateau: Point in recovery when progress slows or stops; often used as criterion for discontinuing therapy services

Posterior fossa: A small space in the skull, found near the brainstem and cerebellum

Postictal: Phase that follows an attack such as acute epilepsy; subjective sensation can be variable

Proprioception: Ability to sense location, movement, and action of parts of the body without visual cuing

Ptosis: Drooping eyelid

Recanalization: Restoration of blood flow to an arterial occlusion site

Spasticity: Unusual tightness, or stiffness, of muscle due to increased tone, or hypertonia; occurs within days to weeks in 30% of stroke patients

Stereognosis: Ability to recognize and identify objects by feeling them

Subcortical: Referring to the area below the cerebrum; predominantly white matter

Sulcus (plural is sulci): Deep grooves on the surface of the cerebral hemisphere

Supratentorial: Refers to portions of the brain above the tentorium; *see* Tentorium

Symmetry: Two sides having the same size and shape

Tentorium: Extension of the dura mater that separates the cerebellum from the inferior portion of the occipital lobes

Thrombectomy: Procedure to remove a blood clot from an artery with image guidance

Thrombolysis: Dissolution, or lysis, of a blood clot

Tonic: Pertaining to, or characterized by, tension or contraction, especially muscular tension

Ventricles: Four hollow spaces in the brain that are filled with cerebrospinal fluid

Vertigo: Sensation of moving around in space, or having objects move around the person; indicates disturbance of the equilibratory apparatus

Wernicke's area: Region in the dominant temporal lobe responsible for comprehension of language

White matter: Bundles of myelinated axons that connect various gray matter areas of the brain and carry nerve impulses between neurons

INDEX

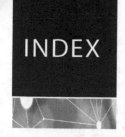

Printed in the United States
by Baker & Taylor Publisher Services